1

SCHIZOPHRENIA EDUCATION GUIDE FOR PATIENTS AND CAREGIVERS

Living With Schizophrenia

By: Edwards H. Benn

ISBN: 9781687759177

Dedication

To the thousands of families who must deal with schizophrenia every day of their lives: your courage, endurance, and hope are a source of inspiration for all.

TABLE OF CONTENTS

Prologue

Until a cure is found, this guide gives the reader: much insight into the challenges that a person recovering from schizophrenia must face; understanding of the disorder itself, its symptoms, treatments, and its impact on families, advice on how to cope with schizophrenia, and information about the service system. Many experts and family members have devoted numerous hours to this project. It is our belief that this reference manual will help to alleviate the suffering caused by schizophrenia — the suffering of those who have it, and their families because the understanding it imparts on you, the reader, will enable you to better cope with the illness.

This book will benefit families, as well as professional caregivers, and the community at large. We can all benefit from a clearer understanding of schizophrenia. The information contained herein has been gathered from many sources, and reviewed by several experts. It is not, however, intended to replace consultation with professionals.

Our roles bring us into contact with numerous families who struggle with schizophrenia, yet devote many volunteer hours of their lives to improve the quality of life for other people. We urge you to come and meet them. Then you too may help alleviate the suffering caused by schizophrenia.

CHAPTER 1: Introduction

Since the first edition of this book, significant progress has been made, particularly in the treatment of schizophrenia. New drug therapies have emerged, and pharmaceutical companies continue to research and develop medications to help battle schizophrenia. The health care field has adopted a comprehensive strategy for helping people with the illness. While drug therapy remains the cornerstone of recovery, psychosocial treatment has a significantly positive impact on the quality of life of persons with schizophrenia. Various programs are available to help people develop their social skills; learn job skills and get jobs; deal with stress and distress in their lives; understand their illness and its impact on their lives, and achieve as functional a recovery as is possible. And all of this can be done in the community, outside the hospital environment. Gone are the days where a hospital is the only place you can turn to. Now, we have Crisis Response Systems, Clubhouses, and Assertive Community Treatment Teams among other emergency, treatment, and rehabilitation services.

Much has been learned about schizophrenia, thanks to ongoing research. Evidence supporting biological cause is abundant, and now points at genetic origin. Gone for good are the days when practitioners blamed parents, and out of guilt, parents blamed themselves.

It is exciting to know that awareness about schizophrenia has improved, and continues to grow, hopefully at an increasing pace. This is important not only for support of research, but also for those who experience the disorder. A better understanding in society helps all those affected – bringing them empathy and compassion, and maybe even saving some lives!

This reference manual extends practical advice based on experience; experience that families have willingly shared for the benefit of readers. They have learned the importance of being armed with knowledge to deal with schizophrenia. It is upon their advice we have chosen various ideas and topics. We hope by reading it, you will have a good start on learning about schizophrenia.

The scope of this publication is broad, and is not meant to replace medical advice. The most important message the contributing families would like to pass on to you is this: schizophrenia is NOT an illness you can deal with on your own. By joining a support group, you can deal more effectively with your community and provincial health care system, establish your rights, and get appropriate help for someone who is ill. Coping with schizophrenia can be easier when you are not struggling alone.

We hope this book will help you with some of the issues and challenges that schizophrenia presents. Topics are broken down for easy digestion and quick reference. As well, subject areas have been separated, for easy reproduction.

Remember – it is only through understanding that you will find true compassion, and the strength to cope! Let us help you, starting with this book!

CHAPTER 2: What Is Schizophrenia?

DEFINING SCHIZOPHRENIA

Schizophrenia is an extremely complex mental disorder: in fact it is probably many illnesses masquerading as one. Symptoms are believed to be caused by a biochemical imbalance in the brain. Recent research reveals that schizophrenia may be a result of misaligned neuronal development in the fetal brain which develops into full-blown illness in late adolescence or early adulthood. The disorder is characterized by delusions, hallucinations, disturbances in thinking and communication, and withdrawal from social activity. Schizophrenia is a serious but treatable brain disorder which affects a person's ability to know what is reality and what is not. A simple explanation of how the brain works helps us to define schizophrenia.

There are billions of nerve cells in the brain. Each nerve cell has branches that transmit and receive messages from other nerve cells. The nerve endings release chemicals, called neurotransmitters, which carry the messages from the end of one nerve branch to the cell body of another. In the brain afflicted with schizophrenia, something goes wrong in this communication system.

In Schizophrenia: Straight Talk for Family and Friends (p. 41), Maryellen Walsh uses the analogy of a telephone switchboard to explain schizophrenia. "In most people the brain's switching system works well. Incoming perceptions are sent along appropriate signal paths, the switching process goes off without a hitch, and appropriate feelings, thoughts, and actions go back out again to the world... in the brain afflicted with schizophrenia... perceptions come in but get routed along the wrong path, or get jammed, or end up at the wrong destination."

The disorder may develop so gradually that it is undetectable in the person for a long time, or it may have a very sudden onset with rapid development. It most commonly strikes between the ages of fifteen and twenty-five years, and has therefore come to be known as Youth's Greatest Disabler. Schizophrenia is found world wide, affecting people of all races, cultures, and social classes; people who are normal and intelligent; people in all walks of life. In Canada one in every one hundred persons is diagnosed with this disorder in their lifetime; over three hundred thousand people in all. Schizophrenia does not discriminate, but occurs in men and women, affecting one percent of the global populace.

Schizophrenia is undoubtedly an intimidating illness; perhaps difficult to grasp at first. Learning as much as you can about the disorder will help you assert as much control as possible over its impact on you, and your family.

CAUSES OF SCHIZOPHRENIA

Sometimes schizophrenia-like symptoms may occur with other diseases such as Huntington's disease, phenylketonuria, Wilson's disease, epilepsy, tumor, encephalitis, meningitis, multiple sclerosis, and numerous other diseases. The real schizophrenia is diagnosed when these other conditions are excluded as the source of psychotic symptoms.

The precise cause of schizophrenia remains unknown. Changes in key brain functions, such as perception, emotions, and behaviour, indicate that the brain is the biological site of schizophrenia. Some researchers suspect neurotransmitters (the substances through which cells communicate) may be involved. There may be changes in dopamine, serotonin, or other neurotransmitters. The limbic system (an area of the brain involved with emotion), the thalamus (which coordinates outgoing messages), and several other brain regions may also be affected.

GENES AND GENETIC RISK

To a large extent, the activity of neurotransmitters is controlled by genes, and there is very strong evidence indicating that genes are involved in causing schizophrenia. This evidence derives from family, twin and other studies. Schizophrenia occurs in 1% of the general population, but the risk is increased if a relative is affected. There is a 10-15% chance of developing the illness when a sibling or one parent has schizophrenia; when both parents have schizophrenia, the risk rises to approximately 40%-50%. Nieces, nephews, or grandchildren of someone with schizophrenia have about a 3% chance of developing the disorder. The chance that an identical twin will be affected with schizophrenia if his/her co-twin has this illness, is about 50%. Genetic counsellors can be helpful in providing risks tailored to the individual's family illness pattern.

No schizophrenia genes have been found yet. However, researchers have identified several regions on the chromosomes where schizophrenia genes are likely to be. In the future, genes may be found which could help in diagnosis and genetic counselling, and eventually in developing more specific treatments for schizophrenia. Genetic subtype: a possible genetic subtype of schizophrenia has recently been identified that is associated with a small deletion (piece missing) on chromosome 22. The 22q Deletion Syndrome likely occurs in a small subset of people with schizophrenia who often have learning disabilities and somewhat nasal speech, and may have congenital heart defects, or other physical abnormalities.

STRESS & INFECTIONS

The role of stress in schizophrenia is unclear. Stress does not cause the illness, but emotional or physical stress (e.g., infections) can trigger or worsen the symptoms when the illness is already present.

DRUG ABUSE

Drugs (including alcohol and street drugs) themselves do not cause schizophrenia. However, street drugs and alcohol can make psychotic symptoms worse if a person already has schizophrenia. Some drugs (amphetamines or phencyclidine/angel dust) can temporarily create schizophrenia-like symptoms in well persons.

NUTRITION

While scientists recognize that proper nutrition is essential for the well being of a person with the illness, they do not agree that a lack of certain vitamins causes schizophrenia. Cures with megavitamin therapy are not proven and are often very expensive. Some people do improve while taking vitamins; however, this may be due to the antipsychotic medication they are taking at the same time, the therapeutic effect of a structured diet, vitamin and medication regime, or they may be part of the 30% who recover no matter what treatment is used. Good nutrition is important to the well being of a person suffering from schizophrenia, but alone can not cure the disease, or lead to a successful recovery.

SCHIZOPHRENIA DEFINITELY IS:

NOT caused by childhood experiences NOT caused by poverty NOT caused by domineering mothers/passive fathers NOT caused by parental negligence, and NOT caused by guilt, failure or misbehaviour.

The more research reveals about the causes of schizophrenia, the better we understand this disorder, and the better modern medicine is able to help us. In research lies hope for a future cure of this illness. And hope begins with you!

PUTTING THE PUZZLE TOGETHER: WHAT IT IS... WHAT IT IS NOT!

SCHIZOPHRENIA IS:

- A brain disease; a biological illness
- Identified by internationally agreed upon and fairly specific symptoms
- Characterized by disorganization of thought/perception
- Characterized by apathy, lack of interest, lack of attention, social withdrawal
- A disorder that often strikes people in their prime (age 15-25 years)
- Recovery depends on treatment

SCHIZOPHRENIA IS NOT:

- Rare – no one is immune
- A split personality
- The result of any action or personal failure by the individual

CHAPTER 3: Recognizing Schizophrenia

SYMPTOMS

Just as other illnesses have signs or symptoms, so does schizophrenia. The symptoms may vary, however, with the individual. Persons with schizophrenia will display symptoms as they struggle to discern reality from their own perceptions. Their level of functioning will deteriorate in areas such as:

- work or academic achievements
- personal care and hygiene
- interaction with others

Personality changes are a key to recognizing schizophrenia. At first, the changes may be subtle, minor, and go unnoticed. As they worsen they become obvious to family members, friends, teachers, and/or co-workers. There is a loss of feelings or emotions, and a lack of interest and motivation. A normally outgoing person may become withdrawn, quiet, moody, suspicious, and/or paranoid. The person may laugh when told a sad story, may cry over a joke, or may be unable to show any emotion at all.

One of the most profound changes is in the ill person's ability to think clearly and logically. Thoughts may be slow in forming, or come extra fast, or not at all. The person may jump from topic to topic, seem confused, or have difficulty reaching easy conclusions. Thinking may be coloured by delusions and false beliefs that resist logical explanations. One person may express strong ideas of persecution, convinced that he/she is being spied on or plotted against. Others may experience grandiose delusions and feel like Superman – capable of anything and invulnerable to danger. Others still may feel a strong religious drive or bizarre mission to right the wrongs of the world.

Perceptual changes turn the world of the ill person topsy-turvey. The nerves carrying sensory messages to the brain from the eyes, ears, nose, skin, and taste buds become confused, and the person sees, hears, smells, and feels sensations which are not real. These are called hallucinations.

It is not difficult to understand why individuals who experience these profound and frightening changes will often seek to keep them secret, deny that anything is happening, or avoid people and situations where they may be discovered. The feedback they receive when they express hallucinations or delusions is disbelief. Ill persons, therefore, feels misunderstood and rejected, and ceases to share their thoughts as a result.

These intense internal experiences trigger other feelings of panic, fear, and anxiety – natural reactions under the circumstances. These feelings can further amplify their extreme emotional state. The psychological burden may be intense: most of it kept inside, its existence denied. The pain of schizophrenia is further accentuated by the persons' awareness of the anguish and suffering they are causing their family and friends.
Those who suffer from schizophrenia require a lot of understanding, patience, and reassurance that they will not be abandoned.

As the symptoms of schizophrenia become noticeable, the ill person will likely experience a sense of alarm and fear. Obviously, the sooner the symptoms are recognized and diagnosed, the sooner the person will benefit from medical help. Once you've confronted the disorder and the fear that goes along with it, you're on your way to recovery.

DEFINING POSITIVE AND NEGATIVE SYMPTOMS

Understanding the terminology used by medical professionals can help you in your efforts to deal with this illness. The symptoms of schizophrenia are classified into two categories: positive symptoms and negative symptoms. They are described for you below:

POSITIVE SYMPTOMS

Hallucinations are thought to be a result of over-sharpening of the senses and of the brain's inability to interpret and respond appropriately to incoming messages. Persons with schizophrenia may hear voices or see visions that are not there, or experience unusual sensations on or in their bodies. Auditory hallucinations, the most common form, involve hearing voices that are perceived to be inside or outside of the person's body. Sometimes the voices are complimentary or reassuring. Sometimes they are threatening, punitive, frightening, and may command the individual to do things that may be harmful.

Delusions are strange and steadfast beliefs that are held only by the person suffering from the disorder. They are maintained despite obvious evidence to the contrary. For example, someone with schizophrenia may interpret red and green traffic signals as instructions from space aliens. Many people with schizophrenia who suffer from persecutory delusions are termed paranoid. They believe that they are being watched, spied upon, or plotted against. A common delusion is that one's thoughts are being broadcast over the radio or television, or that other people are controlling the ill person's thoughts. Delusions are resistant to reason. It is of no use to argue that the delusion is not real.

Thought disorder refers to problems in the way that a person with schizophrenia processes and organizes thoughts. For example, the person may be unable to connect thoughts into logical sequences.

Racing thoughts come and go so rapidly that it is not possible to catch them. Because thinking is disorganized and fragmented, the person's speech is often incoherent and illogical. Thought disorder is frequently accompanied by inappropriate emotional responses: words and mood do not appear connected to each other. The result may be something like laughing when speaking of somber or frightening events. Altered sense of self is a term describing a blurring of the ill person's feeling of whom he/she is. It may be a sensation of being bodiless, or non- existent as a person. The ill individual may not be able to tell where his/her body stops and the rest of the world begins. Or he/she may feel as if the body is separated from the person.

NEGATIVE SYMPTOMS

Lack of motivation or apathy is a lack of energy or interest in life that is often confused with laziness. Because ill persons have very little energy, they may not be able to do much more than sleep and pick at meals. Persons with schizophrenia can be experiencing life without any real interest in it.

Blunted feelings or blunted affect refers to a flattening of the emotions. Because facial expressions and hand gestures may be limited or nonexistent, individuals with schizophrenia seems unable to feel or show any emotion at all. This does not mean that the individuals do not feel emotions and are not receptive to kindness and consideration. They may be feeling very emotional but cannot express it outwardly. Blunted affect may become a stronger symptom as the disease progresses.

Depression involves feelings of helplessness and hopelessness, and may stem in part from realizing that schizophrenia has changed one's life; that the feeling experienced in the psychotic state is an illusion, and that the future looks bleak. Often persons believe that they have behaved badly, destroyed relationships, and are unlovable.

Depressed feelings are very painful and may lead to talk of, or attempts at, suicide. Social withdrawal may occur as a result of depression; a feeling of relative safety in being alone; being caught up in one's own feelings, and/or fearing that one cannot manage the company of others. People with schizophrenia frequently lack an interest in socializing, or at least the ability to demonstrate/express this interest.

EARLY WARNING SIGNS OF ONSET

One of the difficulties in reading the early warning signs of schizophrenia is the easy confusion with some typical adolescent behaviors.
Schizophrenia can begin to affect an individual during the teen years, a time when many rapid physical, social, emotional, and behavioral changes normally occur. There is no easy method to tell the difference. It's a matter of degree. Family members tell of different experiences.
Some sensed early on that their child, spouse, or sibling was not merely going through a phase, a moody period, or reaction to the abuse of drugs or alcohol. Others did not feel their relative's behaviour had been extraordinary. If you have any concerns, the best course of action is to seek the advice of a trained mental health specialist.

The following list of early warning signals of mental illness was developed by families affected by schizophrenia:

Most Common Signs

- Social withdrawal, isolation, and suspiciousness of others
- Deterioration and abandonment of personal hygiene
- Flat expressionless gaze
- Inability to express joy

- Inability to cry, or excessive crying
- Inappropriate laughter
- Excessive fatigue and sleepiness, or an inability to sleep at night (insomnia)

Other Signs

- Sudden shift in basic personality
- Depression (intense and incessant)
- Deterioration of social relationships
- Inability to concentrate or cope with minor problems
- Indifference, even in highly important situations
- Dropping out of activities (and life in general)
- Decline in academic or athletic performance
- Unexpected hostility
- Hyperactivity or inactivity, or alternating between the two
- Extreme religiousness or preoccupation with the occult
- Drug or alcohol abuse
- Forgetfulness and loss of valuable possessions
- Involvement in auto accidents
- Unusual sensitivity to stimuli (noise, light, colour)
- Altered sense of smell and taste
- Extreme devastation from peer or family disapproval
- Noticeable and rapid weight loss
- Attempts at escape through geographic change; frequent moves or hitch-hiking trips
- Excessive writing (or childlike printing) without apparent meaning
- Early signs of migraine
- Fainting
- Irrational statements
- Strange posturing
- Refusal to touch persons or objects; insulation of hands with paper, gloves, etc.

- Shaving head or removal of body hair
- Cutting oneself; threats of self mutilation
- Staring, not blinking, or blinking incessantly
- Rigid stubbornness
- Peculiar use of words or language structure
- Sensitivity and irritability when touched by others
- Change of behaviour: dramatic or insidious

None of these signs by themselves indicate the presence of mental illness. Few of those who helped compile this list said that they had acted on these early warning signs. With the benefit of hindsight, however, these family members urge you to seek medical advice if several of the behaviours listed above are present, or constitute a marked change from previous behaviour, and persist over a few weeks.

Many families noticed that there was no logical flow of ideas during conversation. Others noticed that their relative began speaking out loud to no one, and did not seem to hear other people speaking to him/her. One young man began researching all religions and cults.

Another young man began turning off all radios because he believed that he was receiving messages through this medium. In some families, their relative destroyed his/her bank book, birth certificate, and photographs. Signs of paranoia became apparent in many cases. A relative would begin talking about plots against him/her, and had evidence that he/she was being poisoned. One man said that whenever his wife saw people talking, she assumed they were talking about her.

Eventually, families reached a point where they could not tolerate the differences in behaviour any longer. Many commented that there was much confusion in the home, with some resentment and anger toward the person behaving strangely. Siblings often felt that their brother or sister was merely lazy and shirking responsibilities; children were embarrassed and confused by their parent acting so differently; parents disagreed on how to handle their child's problems; or the stability of the family frequently suffered. All contributors stressed that you should not wait for tensions to reach such extreme levels. You should seek outside help from your family physician or some other appropriate source.

It is important to remember that early diagnosis leads to early treatment, taking you to the path of recovery.

SCHIZOPHRENIA IN CHILDREN & ADOLESCENTS

CHILDHOOD ONSET

Childhood-onset schizophrenia (onset by age 12) is a rare, clinically severe form of schizophrenia that is associated with disrupted linguistic and social development long before the appearance of definitive psychotic symptoms. In its early phases, the disorder is difficult to recognize. Child psychiatrists look for several of the following early warning signs:

- Difficulty discerning dreams from reality
- Seeing things which aren't really there
- Hearing voices which are not real
- Confused thinking
- Vivid and bizarre thoughts and ideas
- Extreme moodiness
- Odd behavior
- Paranoia (thinking people are deliberately trying to harm them)
- Behaving younger than their years
- Severe anxiety and fearfulness
- Not being able to discern television from reality, and/or
- Severe problems with making and keeping friends

Rather than an acute onset, schizophrenia in a child may occur slowly, over a long period of time. You may notice that the child becomes shy or withdrawn when he/she used to enjoy interacting with others. He/she may start talking about strange fears and ideas, or say things that don't make sense. You may notice your child suddenly clinging to you a lot. It may be that the child's teachers notice some of these early signs being exhibited at school. Two of the most commonly reported psychotic features in children are auditory hallucinations and delusions.

DIAGNOSIS

Assessing possible psychosis in a child requires multiple sessions to establish the mental status of the child; details of the child's history including school reports, any neuropsychological test data, speech and language evaluations, and neurological and genetic consultations. If your child is experiencing hallucinations and/or delusions, this evidence alone is insufficient to diagnose schizophrenia. Chronic symptoms and social impairment (e.g., historical developmental problems and changes in academic and social functioning) are key determinants. Researchers feel that the precursor of schizophrenia may include:

- Developmental delays
- Disruptive behaviour disorders
- Expressive and receptive language deficits
- Impaired gross motorfunctioning
- Learning and academic problems
- IQ in the borderline to low-average range
- Transient symptoms of pervasive developmental disorder (autistic-like)

Children who have been diagnosed with schizophrenia should be monitored very closely for several years. As new information
becomes available from observing the child, the diagnosis may need to be reevaluated.

TREATMENT

Children who have been diagnosed with schizophrenia will usually benefit from medication (to diminish their symptoms) and psychosocial treatments. Many issues should be considered in developing a treatment plan including the child's current clinical status, cognitive level, developmental stage, and the severity of the illness. To support the therapeutic relationship with the child, it is important that he/she has a consistent group of caregivers to enable him/her to form a trust in his/her care. At this age, persons with schizophrenia will have difficulty understanding the nature of their illness. It is, therefore, important for parents/guardians and caregivers to know how to recognize changes in mood, behaviour, or thought processes that may indicate relapse in order that treatment can be obtained quickly. Researchers feel that early detection of clinical deterioration is important because psychotic relapses may have a cumulative effect and impede a good recovery level of functioning. Parents should seek counselling on how to recognize the symptoms and behaviours associated with their child's disorder; how to provide the least stressful environment for the child, and problem-solving strategies to deal with disturbing behaviours.

Both typical and atypical neuroleptic drugs are acceptable first-line treatments for children with schizophrenia. Choosing a type of antipsychotic is based on past response, family history of response, cost, and the ill person's tolerance of side effects.

Note that children are susceptible to the same side effects from neuroleptics as are adults. Also, they have a higher vulnerability to side effects such as weight gain, extrapyramidal symptoms, and tardive dyskinesia.

In order to sustain a good recovery, it is best to minimize stress for your ill child. As children recover, they can be integrated back into their environments of home, community, and school. Children with schizophrenia often need individualized school programs and special activities. Strong levels of support from parents and caregivers will be important, especially because of the child's vulnerability to relapse.

Psychosocial interventions applicable to your ill child include occupational therapy that focuses on activities of daily living, social skills training, speech and language therapy, and recreational and art therapy. During the stable phase it is important to monitor the child's cognitive impairments as well as assets. This information can be helpful in planning the child's treatment, and can better prepare him/her for adjustment into adulthood.

If you are concerned, have the child completely evaluated by a psychiatrist. Families recommend that you ask your physician or pediatrician to refer your child to a psychiatrist who is specifically trained to deal with children who have schizophrenia.

There is evidence to suggest that early treatment with antipsychotic medications can prevent detrimental changes that may result from prolonged untreated psychosis.

Facing the possibility that your child might be suffering from schizophrenia is undoubtedly heartbreaking. The best way to help your child and cope with this disorder is to make knowledge your suit of armour, and hope your ally!

ADOLESCENTS WITH SCHIZOPHRENIA

Schizophrenia has its peak onset from approximately age 15-25. Therefore, the first signs of the disorder frequently appear during adolescence. Adolescence is a challenging stage for any family, but when an adolescent is diagnosed with schizophrenia, the challenges become truly daunting.

RECOGNIZING THE SYMPTOMS

Early onset might signal a more severe form of illness, possibly associated with stronger genetic predisposition (family history of schizophrenia), or more premorbid abnormalities (long-standing abnormalities that existed prior to the first onset of symptoms), e.g., learning disorder, pervasive developmental disorder (disorders with autistic-like characteristics), impaired social skills, etc.

While the major symptoms of schizophrenia in adolescents are essentially the same as in adults, it is often difficult in young people to discriminate schizophrenia from affective psychoses (e.g., depression or manic-depression with psychotic features, or schizoaffective disorder). This is because symptoms may appear mixed and undifferentiated in first psychotic episodes in young people. There is, unfortunately, no definitive test for any of these disorders, and the diagnosis relies heavily on observed and reported symptoms. It is therefore difficult
to be one hundred percent certain about the diagnosis in the early stages of illness, especially in children and adolescents, and the diagnosis may be revised in the first few years.

Early onset cases often tend to have a gradual, insidious onset of illness, rather than an abrupt onset. There is often a long period of gradual deterioration in functioning over months or years, referred to as the prodrome, which precedes the onset of overt psychotic symptoms (e.g., delusions, hallucinations, grossly disorganized thinking, and generally being out of touch with reality). The prodrome may be characterized by apathy, withdrawal, speaking less, declining interests and school performance, loss of contact with friends, loss of initiative, bizarre or occult interests/preoccupations, odd behaviours or rituals, neglect of hygiene/grooming, and disorganized thinking manifested as difficulty concentrating or engaging in coherent conversation.

The use of drugs or alcohol may act as a trigger (for an illness that was inevitably going to develop at some point in time), or can signify the adolescent's way of dealing with his/her symptoms (to relieve or mask them). Psychosis that is purely drug or alcohol induced should resolve within days or weeks of not using these substances.

Other possible signs include unruly, antisocial, delinquent-like behaviour, or aggression.

The prodrome may resemble depression, and it may be difficult to distinguish schizophrenia at this early stage, especially since an
adolescent becoming ill with schizophrenia may feel depressed. It is more likely, however, that the ill individual's mood can be described as blunted or flat rather than sad, and there may seem to be an inability to experience or express appropriate emotion at all.

TREATMENT

Acute psychotic episodes, particularly first episodes, usually require hospitalization for a few weeks for assessment and stabilization.
Further treatment can be provided on an outpatient basis in a hospital clinic staffed by a psychiatrist and a nurse. Ill individuals whose course of illness has stabilized, and for whom a medication regime has been established, may be able to receive their treatment from a non-hospital based psychiatrist, family doctor or pediatrician, but many people require re-admissions to hospital for acute psychotic episodes, especially in the first few years.

Sometimes an ill person does not recognize their illness, and refuses treatment. Your province has mental health legislation that will enable you to get help for your ill relative. Consult your provincial Schizophrenia Society, and a mental health or legal professional with expertise in these matters. (See section on Legal Issues, Mental Health Legislation, p. 170 for more information.)

The issues regarding medication treatment for adolescents are much the same as for adults. Certain factors are of added importance in adolescents, such as the need to optimize cognitive (intellectual) functioning (alertness, concentration, memory etc.) as much as possible to facilitate the continuance of academic studies. Certain side effects, such as weight gain and acne, are particularly problematic for adolescents and may lead to non-compliance with treatment.

Compliance is generally a major problem for adolescents, and often requires extra effort on the part of parents to help ensure that their child takes the medication.

A supportive, empathic and stable doctor-patient relationship is naturally important in ensuring compliance with medication, as adolescents with schizophrenia are frequently mistrustful and guarded, if not overtly paranoid, and lack insight about the need for treatment. Once stabilized, the doctor, nurse or other therapist can engage the adolescent in ongoing supportive counselling, talking about day-to-day events and stresses, encouraging the adolescent to verbalize thoughts and feelings and develop better reality-testing and problem-solving abilities. More intensive, introspective, analytically-oriented psychotherapy is generally not applied, as such therapy can be too stressful and disorganizing for individuals with schizophrenia.

COPING WITH YOUR TEENAGER'S ILLNESS

Families usually need a lot of emotional and practical support while coming to terms with their loved one's illness, and steering their way through the turbulent first few years. In many cases the first few years are the worst, and the illness may begin to stabilize thereafter. The diagnosis represents for many parents a devastating loss of ideals and expectations. Understandably, you may go through a grieving process as you struggle to accept the new reality. It is important to know that you could not have caused this brain disorder in your child any more than you could have caused diseases such as Alzheimer's dementia.

Stressful family interactions (e.g., high levels of hostility and criticism) just like other stresses can, however, contribute to relapse of symptoms in individuals who already suffer from schizophrenia.

Families can benefit by receiving as much education as possible about the illness and its management, including information about how to minimize communication/interaction patterns that might cause added stress for all involved. Additional parent support is available in the form of family meetings with a social worker, to address the impact of the illness on the family, and to obtain help in working out the best way to manage the individual's behaviour and communicate effectively with them. Parent and sibling support groups can also be very helpful.

Remember that as family and caregivers, you are part of the solution, not part of the problem. Families have become increasingly empowered in recent years, becoming a most important lobby group, and influencing policy and funding for schizophrenia. Parents should participate in their child's treatment, regularly attending appointments with their child's doctor or nurse, and providing useful information regarding their child's symptoms and functioning (while respecting the adolescent's increasing need for a degree of privacy and autonomy and avoiding infantilizing the adolescent). Relationships with adolescents can be stormy sometimes, as they may vent frustration and anger on the people with whom they feel the most secure.

The needs of siblings should also not be forgotten during the illness. Siblings need love and attention, reassurance and explanations for their mentally ill sibling's behaviour. Please refer to Chapter 10 (2) (ii) for more information on this subject.

DAILY LIVING

Ill persons may need to leave the family home and live in a structured, supervised residential setting such as a group home. This may be

necessary due to behaviour that is too difficult to manage at home, or too disruptive to siblings, or it may be a developmentally appropriate stage in separation from parents and preparation for semi-independent or independent living. Strained family relationships can sometimes improve when mentally ill adolescents and their family have more space and time to themselves, and there is less day-to-day stress in their relationships.

EDUCATIONAL/VOCATIONAL NEEDS

Once ill persons are in the recovery stage, they may be able to continue with academic studies or job training. Adolescents with schizophrenia usually have special educational needs. They may require additional supports and a reduced academic load, or they may benefit from being in an alternative school/day program specifically designed for adolescents suffering or recovering from mental illness. Such schools might be connected to hospital clinics or community mental health agencies.

Older adolescents may need assistance with vocational training, job placement, or post-secondary education, if appropriate. Many will require financial support in the form of a government disability pension whereby part-time work, sheltered employment, or volunteer work may be more suitable for their level of functioning.

SOCIAL NEEDS

Schizophrenia leads to impairment of social skills, loss of initiative, and frequently, paranoia. The result is often active social avoidance. Peer relations are critical to normal adolescent development. Adolescents with schizophrenia may need help in improving their social skills and reconnecting with peer groups. Some adolescents recovering from an acute psychotic episode and hospitalization may be successful at reconnecting with old friends. Others find it easier to relate to peers who have also experienced mental illness. Social reintegration may be assisted by participation in social skills training groups, psychiatric day programs, or structured social activities in the community.

It is important to note that boys often get this illness at an earlier age than girls. The implications of this can be devastating to a young man whose social skills are not yet fine tuned (boys social skills typically develop slower than those of their female counterparts). Since women tend to get the illness at an older age, their social skills are usually developed, and they may have already established relationships with a male partner.

CASE MANAGEMENT SERVICES

Case management services are very helpful in coordinating all the above elements of daily life. A case manager is a community worker assigned to help the mentally ill adolescent and his/her family with a full range of needs in a flexible, community-based manner. The case manager develops a long-term relationship with the individual and his/her family, liaising with mental health services, linking the individual to appropriate services for his/her various needs (e.g., residential, financial, educational, vocational, social) and providing crisis support when necessary. For more information on this subject, please refer to Chapter 8 (3).

OUTLOOK

Schizophrenia is a severe and persistent mental illness, not just a phase, and realistic expectations need to be set in terms of the individual's functioning. But there is much more room for optimism now than in the past. The goal of therapy is not only to help adolescents regain as much as possible of their previous level of functioning, but also to help them to progress with the develop-mental tasks appropriate to their age. Therapy needs to take into account the individual needs of adolescents, with their uniquely evolving personality, and particular home and social circumstances. With early and continuing treatment (antipsychotic medication and psychosocial rehabilitation), and ongoing research to improve treatments, adolescents with schizophrenia may be able to achieve significantly better functioning than was the case in the past for

many people suffering from this serious illness. ●

CHAPTER 4: Diagnosing Schizophrenia

OTHER SIMILAR ILLNESSES

There is, as yet, no simple lab test to diagnose schizophrenia. Therefore, the diagnosis is based on symptoms — what the person says, what the family reports, and what the doctor observes.

To reach a diagnosis of schizophrenia, other possible causes such as drug abuse, epilepsy, brain tumor, thyroid or other metabolic disturbances, such as hypoglycemia, as well as other physical illnesses that have symptoms like schizophrenia, must be ruled out. The condition must also be clearly differentiated from bipolar (manic- depressive) disorder. Some ill individuals show symptoms of both schizophrenia and manic depression. This condition is termed schizoaffective disorder.

If your doctor does diagnose schizophrenia, do not assume that he/she has ruled out the possibility of another illness. Do not hesitate to ask about other illnesses and ask on what grounds the doctor has determined that schizophrenia is the problem. Where an illness as confusing and variable as schizophrenia is concerned, you should ask for a second medical opinion and a psychiatric referral, whether or not you are satisfied with your doctor's response. A request of this nature is perfectly acceptable. Do not feel that the doctor will take it as a personal criticism.

Caution is in order because seemingly telltale symptoms, even in combination, may not be evidence of schizophrenia. They might be evidence only of an overworked imagination or extreme stress due, for example, to a death in the family, or break-up of a marriage. The crucial factor is the relative ability to turn off the imagination. Today, increasingly precise diagnosis helps to ensure that warning signs are not misinterpreted.

A diagnosis that confirms schizophrenia may be heart- breaking for you and your family. Remember there are many others like you, who have experienced the feelings that burden you. Seek consolation and support at this difficult time. It will help you cope, and you will learn valuable lessons to help the person with schizophrenia.

SEEKING MEDICAL ATTENTION

Family members will likely be the first to recognize the need to get medical attention for he/she affected loved one. Take the initiative. Ask your family doctor for an assessment if mental illness is suspected. It is important to realize that your relative may be genuinely unaware of the abnormality of his/her symptoms — remember that ill persons believe that the hallucinations, delusions, or other symptoms are real. They may, therefore, resist any suggestion to see a physician. Even if ill persons are aware that something is wrong with them, their confusion and fear about the problem may convince them to deny its existence or abnormality.

Efforts to have your relative agree to visit a doctor will likely be more successful when made without reference to strange behaviour (e.g., "You've been acting really weird lately", or any reference to the feelings of others; "Your behaviour has been upsetting this family"). Encouraging the ill person to seek medical attention based on symptoms such as insomnia, lack of energy, or sadness will more likely be perceived as helpful and non-threatening. If your relative agrees to see a doctor, ask the receptionist for a double booking (most appointments are only 10 or 15 minutes long) so that you will not feel rushed. Then, after you have arranged the appointment, send the doctor a letter outlining your concerns as clearly as possible. In addition to assisting the doctor, this will help you be clear about what has been happening. The following is a sample letter:

Dear Dr. Smith,

I have made an appointment for my daughter, Jane, to see you on Monday, May 8, at 10:00 a.m.

Three months ago, Jane began acting in an unusual manner. The following are some of the behaviours that our family has noticed: she cannot sleep at night; has dropped out of her favourite   activities; refuses to see any friends; cries two to three hours a day, and will not allow anyone to touch her.

I have enclosed copies of her last two school reports, and a list of comments made by her friends. I believe that a medical assessment is necessary, and I am anxious to hear your opinion.

Sincerely,

Jane's Mother and/or Father

If your relative refuses to see a physician, however, you should still make an appointment and go on your own. Again, make a double booking, and send a variation of the above letter. After you have visited with the doctor, you may find it easier to get your relative to agree to an appointment.

If you have succeeded in convincing your ill family member to go to the doctor, you need to be aware that this first visit may not resolve anything or answer any questions. Families who have been through this admitted that they had hoped this doctor's visit would be the cure-all, and were frustrated when nothing seemed to happen.

During a doctor's appointment, ill persons may not exhibit the behaviour that you have seen. Some people find talking to a doctor very stressful, and many people with schizophrenia have said that they found themselves going blank during the visit.

However, many people with schizophrenia also said that their fear of going to the doctor was somewhat alleviated when the doctor was able to ask the right questions. Because of the letter received in advance, the doctor was able to focus on the symptoms that were bothering the ill person, and the individual found that he or she was more willing to open up to the doctor. For example, people found it comforting if the doctor said something like: "I understand you've been crying a lot lately. You must feel very confused about this." It is important that you are prepared to supply information to the physician and/or psychiatrist to help them make an assessment.

IF THE ILL PERSON REFUSES TO SEE A PHYSICIAN

If the ill person refuses to go to a doctor's office, you could try to arrange for a house visit by the doctor. If a physician does agree to visit the ill person at home, try to prepare your relative ahead of time. Encourage him/her to cooperate as best you can, but understand that the ill person may still refuse to talk to the doctor. If you cannot arrange for a home visit by a physician, or are having trouble getting the ill person to talk to a doctor, seek assistance from your local mental health clinic. They may be able to direct you to alternative options (e.g., a mobile crisis response team, an assertive community treatment team, etc.).

After you have unsuccessfully exhausted all available avenues for a voluntary physical/mental examination by a psychiatrist or physician, you may consider having a compulsory examination ordered by a judge. All provinces in Canada have mental health legislation provisions that allow any person to apply to a judge for the compulsory psychiatric examination of another person. Mental health laws require that if you request such an order, evidence must be provided to the court that shows the ill person is suffering from a mental disorder, is refusing to see a physician, and meets criteria for harm, danger, or safety concerns as specified by the provincial legislation. If you have kept records (see Keeping Records section below), it is a good idea to offer them to the judge, as they may be helpful to the decision process. Since the procedures and criteria for these court orders differ between provinces, it is advisable to seek assistance from a mental health professional or lawyer who has expertise in these matters. Your provincial Schizophrenia Society may also be able to help you.

If a court order for examination is granted, it is usually the police who take the ill person to a physician. A medical examination is performed to determine if involuntary admission to hospital is warranted under provisions of the provincial mental health legislation.

If the ill person refuses to see a doctor during a crisis that involves violence or endangerment, and the police get involved, the police are authorized by provincial Mental Health Acts to take the ill individual to a hospital or physician for examination. The physician then decides whether or not the ill person will be admitted to a clinic or hospital on an involuntary basis (see the section on Police Involvement,

TIPS ON OBTAINING MEDICAL HELP
(from a family member)

The assessment and treatment of schizophrenia should involve experts in schizophrenia. Consult with your family physician or psychiatrist before accepting any unusual treatment or changing your current treatment program. If you have questions or lack confidence in the advice you receive, remember that you have the right to seek another opinion from another psychiatrist, locally or elsewhere.

When seeking a specialist, you will want someone who is medically competent, who has an interest in the disorder, and who has empathy with people who experience it. More specifically, you will want assistance from a psychiatrist who:

- believes schizophrenia is a biological disorder

- takes the time to do a detailed history

- screens for symptoms/problems that could be related to another illness

- prescribes antipsychotic drugs with due caution and care

- reviews medications and the case regularly

- is interested in the ill individual's entire welfare and makes appropriate referrals for aftercare, housing, social support and financial aid

- involves the family in the treatment process

- explains the ill person's status fully and clearly

Anyone who tells you that schizophrenia does not exist, or that you should avoid medical treatment if you have it, is not acting in your best interests. Also, individuals who offer guaranteed treatments and cures must be regarded with extreme caution.

The world of medicine is strategic to the recovery of people with schizophrenia. Explore it diligently, and get the best it has to offer. The ill person needs and deserves the best, and so do you!

KEEPING RECORDS

When you start seeking medical attention for the ill person, it is important to begin, and maintain, a diary or record of your relative's illness, noting his/her behaviour patterns, any treatment he/she undergoes, and all the steps you have taken to help your relative.

Although this may require considerable effort, experienced family members strongly emphasize the value of record keeping. It will greatly assist you in relaying history to the attending physician(s) and other caregivers, in keeping symptoms and issues organized in your thoughts; as well as being a useful reference should relapse occur.

Records also provide useful information to help a physician or a judge make decisions regarding involuntary hospital admission.

The record should be clear, precise, and in point form. Avoid vague words and rambling descriptions. Medical practitioners stress the importance of listing behaviours that can be observed and measured. For example, you are noting a particular behaviour if you say that Joe refuses to wash, and wears the same clothes every day. This is more useful than saying that Joe looks scruffy. It is also more useful to tell the doctor that Susan cries every night for at least one hour, than to tell the doctor that Susan seems so sad lately. Write down the details of the noted behaviour, and include the day, time and duration, if applicable. Keep a record of your appointments with your doctor, and keep copies of all correspondence.

It is essential that you treat your record as a confidential document, one that should be used with discretion. If your relative has paranoid tendencies, knowledge of your record may only convince him/her that you are spying. On the other hand, some families have found that it is helpful to have their relative's involvement in the record keeping. If you feel it is appropriate, encourage your relative to jot down his/her thoughts and feelings.

You may think that record keeping is just another thorn in your side. The benefit, however, is not only practical but somewhat therapeutic. By documenting important information, you are relieving yourself of the burden to remember.

INITIAL ASSESSMENT

(source: Canadian Clinical Practice Guidelines for the Treatment of Schizophrenia)

The initial assessment of the ill individual should include both a physical examination, and a clinical investigation by a psychiatrist. Generally speaking, a person with a normal health history will undergo tests such as a drug screen, general chemistry screen, complete blood count, and urinalysis. Brain imaging scans may be ordered if neurological signs or symptoms of other brain diseases are present. Neurocognitive testing should be performed. Measurements of intelligence, memory, attention, command functions, language, and visual and motor skills can reveal both preserved and impaired mental abilities — indicating functionality at the community level (and perhaps guiding rehabilitation plans).

The psychiatrist should make specific inquiries relating to the following:

• Positive, negative, and disorganized symptoms, and changes in functioning

• When the psychotic symptoms began and possible precipitating factors (e.g., substance use/abuse)

• Substance use/abuse

• Any history of suicidal thinking and behaviour

• Any history of violence, verbal or physical

• The ill person's general medical history

• Any family history of schizophrenia and other psychotic disorders (including treatment received), other psychiatric disorders (including addictions and suicidal behaviour), and inherited medical illnesses

• The current lifestyle of the individual, including housing environment, finances, social network and activities, work environment, and general functionality in the community

• A developmental history, including social and academic functioning, both in childhood and adolescence

These questions will give the psychiatrist clues to, for example, the potential outcome of treatment (the longer the duration of untreated psychosis, the greater the likelihood of poorer results); whether and where the ill person should be hospitalized; and whether other biological investigations should be performed.

Arming yourself with knowledge is the best way to help you and your relative, as well as the medical experts with whom you will be working. Asking questions of your psychiatrist(s) is not only a reasonable approach to participating in the ill individual's assessment, it is necessary to satisfy yourself with information. A good health professional will expect this.
Do not be afraid to exhibit your concerns, and demonstrate your commitment – the role you play entitles you to the knowledge that will help you deal with this disorder. Here are some questions to which you (regardless of confidentiality issues) are entitled to have answered by the psychiatrist:

Be prepared: Make yourself a list of questions ahead of time. Make sure you have all the answers you want.

Don't be intimidated — the physician's role is to serve you and the ill person!

• What is your diagnosis?

• If your current evaluation is a preliminary one, how long will it take to ascertain a definite evaluation?

• What is the medical cause of this illness?

• Do you feel confident that the possibility of other illnesses has been ruled out?

• Has a neurological examination been conducted? What tests were performed, and what were the results?

• Are there any additional tests that you would recommend at this point in time?

• Would you recommend an independent psychiatric or other specialist's opinion at this point in time?

• What kind of treatment program do you suggest? How will it work, and what are the results we should expect?

• Will other health professionals be involved in this program? If so, how can we ensure their services will be coordinated?

• To whom can we refer our questions or problems when you are not available?

• Do you plan to include psychosocial rehabilitation in the treatment program?

• What will your role/contribution to the treatment process be?

• How often will the ill person be seen by health caregivers, and how long will the sessions be?

• How soon before signs of progress will be evident? What will be the best evidence that the ill individual is responding to the treatment program?

• How much access will the family have to the health caregivers involved?

• What do you see as the family's role in this treatment program?

• What medication(s) are you proposing (ask for name and dosage level)? What is the biological effect of this medication? What are the risks and side effects associated with it? How soon will we know its effectiveness? How will we know it is working? What will it ultimately accomplish?

• Are there other medications that might be appropriate? Why do you prefer this one?

• Are you currently treating other people with schizophrenia?

• When are the best times to contact you? Where is the best place to reach you?

• How familiar are you with support groups and agencies that can help us? How do you monitor medications (e.g., regular blood tests)? What symptoms indicate that a change in dose may be required? Will you be monitoring for depression? How do we ensure medication is taken on a daily basis? How often will you reassess the ill person? How do you reassess the individual?

• What can we do to help you during the treatment process? If hospitalization is required at some point, which hospital do you suggest? What is the best way to ensure the family will be included in plans to discharge the ill person from the hospital? What are the laws about committal and compulsory treatment? What is your philosophy on them?

• Do you have any suggestions about dealing with psychotic episodes? Who do I turn to in the event of an emergency or crisis?

If your relative has manic or depressive symptoms, you might ask the psychiatrist whether a thyroid screening was done, and if not, would it be appropriate to do one? If the ill person is over the age of forty, you will want to understand the physical implications of medications. What effect do they have on cardiac functioning? Should regular electrocardiograms be performed? Has the ill person's blood sugar been measured? Is there any risk of diabetes? Have tests been done to assess other medical problems? See Chapter 9 on Medical Comorbidity of Schizophrenia, p. 112 for more information on health

risks for people with schizophrenia. ●

Once again, be sure to keep a record of all your questions and the responses. You'll be happy to have it as a reference source.

CHAPTER 5: Early Intervention

DEFINITION AND BARRIERS

Early intervention refers to the recognition of the onset of psychosis* (either prodromal stage or first episode of psychosis), and the immediate response to it. We already know from Chapter 3 some of the early signs of onset of schizophrenia. They include, but are not limited to, the following:

- a decrease in functionality

- frequent changes in jobs or places of residence

- changes in personality (e.g., an outgoing teenager becomes withdrawn and avoids opportunities to socialize)

- paranoia (perception of being prosecuted or the subject of attention by media)

- apathy (lack of emotion or interest)

- excessive fatigue and desire to sleep

- insomnia

- depression and/or anxiety

- difficulty with concentration or thinking clearly

- decline in academic, athletic, or work performance

- restlessness or uneasiness

- alcohol or other substance abuse, and/or

- unexpected hostility

These symptoms tend to precede the onset of schizophrenia, and are known as the early course of schizophrenia. Hallucinations, delusions, and/or thought disorder are examples of psychosis, or the acute stage of schizophrenia.

*Please note that psychosis is not only a symptom of schizophrenia, but appears in other serious mental disorders as well.

There are three major hurdles to early intervention. The first is recognition that there is a problem. Studies of ill people experiencing their first episode of psychosis have demonstrated that they typically remain undiagnosed and untreated for several years.[3] Fear and a sense of helplessness may trigger an avoidance type of reaction by the ill person and the family. For example, parents may dismiss the ill person's behaviour as being that of a normal teenager. Another reaction might be to blame the behaviour on a perceived problem with alcohol or other substance abuse. It may be that the ill person senses that he/she is experiencing something out of the ordinary, but does not want others to know about it. It may also be that the ill person does not realize that he/she is experiencing anything unusual. For example, if the ill person is having delusions, he/she likely believes the delusion is reality.

Unfortunately, failure to recognize the problem means that the ill person will likely not seek help until the illness reaches an acute stage. While this lack of acceptance and commitment to do something about the problem is understandable, it becomes the second major hurdle to early intervention. Without treatment, the illness cannot be addressed. Without acceptance, treatment is unlikely to occur. In many cases the ill person can continue to function (e.g., in academic, athletic, or career roles) for years while experiencing symptoms of psychosis, and therefore may choose not to seek treatment until such time as he/she can no longer function.

Once help is sought out, getting access to care and treatment is the third hurdle to early intervention. This third hurdle is attributable to a lack of education, awareness, and expertise within the health care system. Understanding of mental illness and its symptomatology is key to proper assessments, diagnoses, and effective treatment of
schizophrenia. Research indicates that most people with schizophrenia consult a health care practitioner several times before an accurate diagnosis is made and treatment initiated. This policy of waiting for
a complete and accurate diagnosis before commencing treatment is problematic since the process can take up to a year, during which time the ill person continues to suffer.

Poor communication is a component of the access to treatment barrier. The ill person may not be able to adequately express his/her feelings and experiences, leaving a physician with the wrong impression, or at least impeding the diagnostic process. Also, families and ill individuals complain that when they learned of the illness, little or no information about the diagnosis, treatment, and available support was communicated to them by health care professionals. This could be due to the ill person's inability to process the information while unstable, meaning that the timing of communication was inappropriate. It could also be that the manner in which the communication was made did not suit the recipient, so delivery of information was not successful.

Another factor could be insufficient family involvement, caused by the confidentiality issue and failure to get the ill person's permission to divulge information. The danger of insufficient information is twofold. The first problem is it prevents ill people and their families from getting the help and information they need to deal with the diagnosis. The second danger is it may lead to the development of unrealistically high, or overly pessimistic, expectations for the ill person's recovery.

Not all people with schizophrenia have classic textbook symptoms. Every person's experience is unique. If you notice strange and unusual behaviour in your loved one, he/she may need help. It is advisable to consult a health practitioner with mental health expertise immediately.

RATIONALE AND BENEFITS

Research tells us that one of the biggest obstacles to a good recovery from schizophrenia is the length of time the illness has existed before treatment commences. Statistics show that only twenty to thirty percent of people with schizophrenia experience good recoveries.

These statistics have not improved in accordance with the availability of psychosocial support and the advances in antipsychotic therapies. The problem is that before the ill person is treated for the illness, he/she is at risk of losing important skill sets such as social and occupational skills. This is particularly true for adolescent individuals who are in the crucial period of maturation, when much psychological and social development occurs. It is also likely that the ill person's relationship with family will be strained, and his/her pursuit of education or employment interrupted. While medication addresses psychotic symptoms, once these skill sets are lost the ill person will continue to experience a decrease in functioning, resulting in a poorer quality of life, and possibly making the ill person more prone to suicide, depression, aggression, substance abuse, anxiety disorders, and cognitive impairment.

It is also more likely that an ill person will be open to treatment and insight into the illness while still in the early stages of it. Once the positive symptoms (e.g., delusions) have progressed, it is more difficult to engage the ill person in treatment.[4] The earlier in the illness ill persons get interventions, the easier it is to minimize the resulting disability they experience. Long durations of untreated psychosis have been associated with:

Slower and incomplete recoveries More biological abnormalities More

relapses, and Overall poorer long-term outcomes.

SCIENTIFIC DATA:

In February 2000, the Australian and New Zealand Journal of Psychiatry reported results of a study of early psychosis patients and chronic schizophrenia patients. The study revealed that more people who were treated early on in their illness were able to survive in the community for longer than twelve months, than those people whose illness had reached a chronic stage.[5] The analysis was based on their social and occupational functioning and living skills.

The Doctor's Guide News of London, England reported in November 2000 that brain imaging studies performed at the London Institute of Psychiatry showed that substantial changes in the brain are present at the earliest stages of schizophrenia. The changes in the brain actually precede the appearance of psychosis, so that by the time people show signs of psychosis, their brain structures have already changed.
Dr. Tonmoy Sharma, who led the study, suggests that brain imaging may identify characteristics of schizophrenia early enough that immediate treatment could perhaps prevent psychosis and the full development of the illness, and give the ill person a better chance of recovery. The report acknowledges that people with schizophrenia have a better chance of recovery if their psychosis is treated early on in the illness.

In November 2002, the National Library of Medicine reported incidental radiological findings on brain magnetic resonance imaging (MRI) in first-episode psychosis and chronic schizophrenia. The findings show that patients with chronic schizophrenia were more likely to have clinically significant abnormal scans than patients with first- episode psychosis.[7]

Recent developments in research suggest that immediate treatment of the emerging positive symptoms of schizophrenia can greatly reduce the duration of illness, the severity of symptoms, and the impact on the family and community.[8] Early intervention (treatment received immediately after the first episode of psychosis, or during the prodromal phase) contributes to better recoveries. Both the Prevention and Early Intervention Program for Psychosis (London, Ontario) and Early Psychosis Prevention and Intervention Centre (Australia) programs (see Best Early Intervention Practices, p. 63) report that ill individuals who receive appropriate treatment within six months of the onset of psychosis, experience better recoveries than those whose treatment was delayed for more than six months.[9]

The motivation for early intervention is to reduce suffering for those who are ill and their families. The benefits of immediate treatment are encouraging:

- Less interruption in the life of the ill person

- Less strain on the ill person's family

- Greater chance of reintegration into social activities, academic and/or career pursuits

- Reduced chance of suicide

- Less chance of chronic illness (frequent relapses) and disabling disorders (depression, alcohol or substance abuse, anxiety), and

- Overall better functioning and quality of life

THE NEED FOR PUBLIC EDUCATION

Recognizing and accepting that a problem exists, and seeking help are the first steps to receiving treatment for schizophrenia. But how is a person to know that what he/she is experiencing is not something to run and hide from – but rather something that should be treated, sooner rather than later? If and when they do seek medical assistance, how can people suffering symptoms of schizophrenia be sure they will get an appropriate response? The best answer is increased public education and awareness, and better training of health professionals. Public education should be targeted to: authoritative figures in an adolescent's world; to the medical care system; to families with a history of schizophrenia (whose children are at greater risk of developing the disorder); to young people who

exhibit symptoms
of alcohol or substance abuse, and to the general public. Family physicians should have specific training to help them detect mental illness in its early stages. Emergency care units and mental health units of hospitals should have specific training in not only recognizing the early symptoms of schizophrenia, but also minimizing the trauma of a first episode of psychosis for the ill person.

Often times the onset of illness comes at a young age (between ages of fifteen and twenty-five). Young people are typically still dependent on parents, teachers, athletic coaches, guidance counsellors, clergy, youth agencies and others for direction in their lives. These people can be influential in a young person's life, and it is very important that they receive information on mental illness, and the early signs of its onset. Awareness will improve the chance of recognition, and once suspected, a teacher or other figure of authority and influence may help the ill person to accept the problem and seek treatment. If the ill person has a good relationship with a teacher or family doctor, wherein he/she trusts the professional, and feels treated with respect and concern, then there is a good chance that this figure of authority will be one of the first points of contact for the youth. It is essential that such individuals be educated about the warning signs of mental illness, and about taking a distressed young person's complaints seriously. The person with schizophrenia is more likely to seek help voluntarily with the help of someone knowledgeable about mental illness with whom he/she enjoys a healthy interpersonal relationship.

Such a relationship can also contribute to an ongoing treatment plan, if the professional is diligent in maintaining contact with the ill person, offering encouragement and support where appropriate.

Once ill persons embark on the pathway to care, the experiences they have will impact their recovery. Thus it is equally important that doctors and other gatekeepers (nurses, social workers, therapists, paramedics etc.) of the health care system respond adequately and appropriately to an ill person's request for help. Lack of information leads to delays in treatment, which in turn prolongs the suffering for the ill person. The trauma of a first episode of psychosis can be exacerbated by: being treated in an unsuitable environment (e.g., a dismal and dreary psychiatric ward with seriously ill people); by not getting meaningful human attention; by not getting sufficient follow-up and support from community services, and by the stigma attached to mental illness (which comes from lack of education and awareness). While hospitalization is necessary in some cases, much treatment can begin in outpatient clinics or through outreach programs. Gatekeepers need to be aware of available sources of treatment in their community, as well as have up-to date knowledge and training specific to the needs of both ill individuals and their families dealing with schizophrenia (e.g., young people usually require lower doses of medication for effective treatment of psychosis).

The emergency ward is often where a person suffering an episode of psychosis will go. There is a need for emergency wards to have mental health teams with expertise in assessing early psychosis. Gatekeepers should also have referral networks in order that ill individuals do not get lost in the medical system, but are closely followed by the appropriate practitioners. If an ill person's first contact with treatment is severely negative, he/she is not likely to want to remain in the care of the medical system. There is also the risk that the ill individual will suffer post-traumatic stress disorder.

Many ill people and their families report being shocked and angry by the traumatic and stigmatizing experience of hospitalization. Their message is that forcible confinement, isolation, discouraging psychiatric ward environments, and insensitive treatment are far too overwhelming for a young person, and sometimes have more long-term ill effects than the actual experience with psychosis. Young people with schizophrenia need lots of human contact, reassurance, encouragement, counselling, and support to accept their illness.

One of the advantages of having an educated public is that it is easier for the ill person and his/her family to engage the support of their community. If schools and teachers understand the illness, then they can help the young ill person as he/she tries to continue studies. If work environments have a good awareness of mental illness, they are more likely to support an ill person who tries to continue his/her career pursuits. Community support is key to reintegration of the ill individual, and should be engaged as soon as the ill individual is stable – it is counter-productive to prevent an ill person from doing activities he/she is capable of until a firm diagnosis is made (since that can take one or more years). Families will also need hands-on support from their community. They may require respite services, and are likely to need the help and understanding of other relatives and friends. People generally want to be helpful to those in need, and public education fosters the ability of the general public to respond appropriately to schizophrenia, while removing the stigma attached to it.

THE NEED FOR PATIENT AND FAMILY EDUCATION

In 1998 an early intervention survey performed by the Canadian Mental Health Association, British Columbia Division, found that the majority of people with mental illness received either minimal or no information about their diagnosis, or about the treatment and support available to them. The findings cited several problems with education for ill people: inability to process or accept the information at an acute stage of illness; lack of opportunities for education beyond the hospital environment; reluctance of professionals to diagnose based on a first experience; delivery of information failing to successfully and accurately communicate to the recipient (invoking unnecessary fear and serious misunderstandings), and failure of communication to be fitting and sensitive to the recipient (invoking fear, demoralization,
or denial). The study also found that one of the best sources of information was peer-based education, because it provided knowledge in a less threatening manner, and enabled people with mental illness to share experiences with other people in similar situations. It is imperative that ill individuals receive sufficient and appropriate

information and education about schizophrenia in order to foster their acceptance of the illness, a sense of control over it, and a sense of hope for recovery.[11] Education for people with schizophrenia and their families directly impacts the treatment process – without an understanding of the illness, ill people are less likely to fully participate in a proper treatment plan, and families are less likely to know how to help the ill person.

The survey found that while families tend to receive some information during the first episode of illness, it isn't sufficiently specific or practical to help them cope with their situations. Factors such as confidentiality, failure to ask the ill person's permission, resistance to the diagnosis, and lack of assertiveness and understanding of the significant role family members play in helping the ill individual cope with the illness are possible contributors to lack of family education. The danger of insufficient and non-specific information is that families may develop expectations for their ill loved one that are either overly morbid or unrealistically high. Families reported that most information they received was through their own initiative as opposed to a proactive approach by the health care system to involve them. Families need education that is inclusive of all members, and is sensitive to their reaction to the illness. They need counselling and support to help them accept the devastation associated with schizophrenia, and to help them contribute both emotionally and practically to their ill loved one's recovery. They require help in knowing how to communicate with the ill person about the illness. Families also have a need to learn from other families in similar situations, and to have a sense of being understood by others.

EARLY INTERVENTION STRATEGIES

WHAT TO LOOK FOR IN ASSESSMENTS

An individual exhibiting signs of onset of illness or full-blown psychosis should be immediately and rapidly assessed by a physician. Ideally, the ill person should be assessed in a setting that is non-threatening, and that minimizes stigmatization. Examples of such environments include the young person's own home, the office of his/her family physician,

or a community clinic with mental health experts specifically trained to handle these delicate situations.

There are two components to a full and proper assessment for mental illness: the psychosocial component and the physical component. The health practitioner should be asking questions about the ill person's social relationships, school or work performance, recreational pursuits, ability to manage finances, attention to hygiene and clothing, religious activities, interaction with family members and/or others in the home environment, and attention to housework. Your ill relative should also be assessed on his/her current strengths and intact functionality (e.g., academic standing, athletic abilities, job abilities, social abilities) in order that clinicians can target treatment to support the ill person's existing capabilities. Cognitive and intellectual functions should be assessed using a mental status exam. This measures the stressors in the ill individual's life, his/her coping abilities, type of personality, and attitude toward the disorder. Functions should be closely monitored for any changes and the rate at which change takes place. The ill person's medical records (from birth and through the developing years) should be examined. He/She should also be given a complete psychiatric assessment, including details on academic, occupational, recreational, and social history.

The ill person should also undergo basic neurological and general physical examinations prior to engaging in drug therapy. Any movement abnormalities the ill person may have should be determined. Urinalysis along with a complete blood count should be taken in order to help reveal any infections that may be in the body. The ill person should be measured for levels of glucose and electrolytes, and be tested for functioning of the liver, kidneys, and thyroid. He/She should be tested for HIV and sexually transmitted diseases. A toxicology screen (checks the body for poisonous substances) should be taken. Heart function should be assessed. Also, the ill person's weight and body mass index should be measured.

It is essential that any existing medical problems be fully investigated, as they could contribute to more severe psychoses, leading to depression and a greater likelihood of attempts at suicide.

It is recommended that your ill relative undergo diagnostic reassessments several times each year, in accordance with diagnostic criteria checklists or DSM-IV. This will help prevent the possibilities of misunderstandings surrounding the diagnosis, and the chance of having unrealistic expectations. Re-examinations will also help to ensure the ill person is given the appropriate treatment to help him/her recover.

Thorough psychosocial and physical assessments should provide information that will give the ill individual and his/her family as clear a picture as possible on the status of the illness and its impact to date. This will help the ill person and family members to develop realistic expectations for the ill person's recovery. Also, the more complete the assessments, the better able the physician is to prescribe treatment that suits the particular circumstances of the ill individual.

SEVEN PRINCIPLES OF TREATMENT

The purpose of drug therapy and psychosocial treatment for schizophrenia is to help the ill person recover to as near to a normal quality of life as possible. Without treatment, there is little or no chance of recovery. It is important for family members to be aware of ways to help ensure the ill person gets the full benefit of a treatment plan, and adheres to it as prescribed. The following principles of treatment will help to promote a successful recovery:

7 PRINCIPLES OF TREATMENT

1)   The development of a strong and enduring relationship with the treatment team

2)   Attention to the comfort of the ill person

3)   Comprehensive and individualized treatment

4)   Ongoing intensive treatment for at least several years following the first episode of psychosis

5)   Age – and stage – appropriate treatment

6)   Attention to the pace and timing of reintegration

7)   Early family involvement[13]

Development of a strong and enduring relationship with the treatment team.

Surveys of patients and families tell us that a good relationship with one or more members of the treatment team promotes long-term adherence to the treatment plan. If the ill person trusts someone involved in his/her therapy, and feels comfortable approaching and confiding in the practitioner, he/she is more likely to follow the prescribed treatment.

Attention to the comfort of the ill person.

When someone experiences psychosis, it is very distressing. The response he/she receives while undergoing the acute episode of schizophrenia could make the situation worse. If the ill individual is traumatized when hospitalized; experiences poor and confusing assessments; or if he/she suffers strong side effects from drug therapy, then it is less likely the ill person will want to participate in treatment.

Comprehensive and individualized treatment.

Antipsychotic medication and psychosocial therapy coupled together make the best recipe for a complete recovery plan. Every individual is unique, and people with schizophrenia should have individualized treatment plans designed to meet their particular needs and goals, support their strengths, address their weaknesses, and help them maintain a good

46

level of self-esteem and functionality. The goals of treatment should include:

•   The improvement of psychotic symptoms

•   The reintegration of the ill person to his/her normal roles and environments as quickly and effectively as possible

•   The prevention of depression, anxiety and other secondary symptoms

•   The support and improvement of the ill person's self-esteem and capabilities, and

•   The maximization of the ill person's quality of life

Ongoing intensive treatment for at least several years following the first episode of psychosis.

Most people who suffer an acute episode of schizophrenia will take antipsychotic medication for the rest of their lives. It is important that antipsychotic treatment be continuous, as interruptions may lead to a relapse. If the ill person frequently stops treatment, he/she is less likely to make a complete recovery. Psychosocial therapy should also be ongoing and intensive, for at least several years after the first episode of psychosis, in order to support adherence to drug therapy, and promote a complete recovery.

Adolescent individuals need help if a transfer of health care services is required when they reach adulthood. The family should be advised well in advance if services will cease at a certain age, in order to arrange for continuing alternative care.

Age – and stage – appropriate treatment.

It is important that both medication and psychosocial interventions be tailored to the age of the ill individual, as well as to his/her stage in life. For example, young people require lower doses of antipsychotic medicine to maintain stability. Students will need different services than people who are pursuing careers. A female's medication will likely need to be changed if she decides to bear children. Treatment needs to fit the ill person's needs and goals as he/she progresses through life.

Attention to the pace and timing of reintegration.

A primary goal of early intervention is getting the ill person reintegrated into his/her social, occupational, scholastic, athletic, domestic, and other roles as soon as possible. It is important that the plan for reintegration be sensitive to the ill person's ability to cope. If done too quickly, reintegration may cause the ill individual to be overwhelmed and possibly suffer a relapse. Failure to reintegrate successfully will also likely have a negative impact on the person's confidence and self-esteem. The timing and pace of reintegration to each former or new activity must be carefully handled.

Early family involvement.

The concept of early intervention suggests that family members should be involved as early and as fully as possible. They should be educated about the illness, and the importance of their participation in the treatment plan should be emphasized. It is also important that disruption to the family unit be minimized. Chapter 9 deals with the role of the family as well as helping family members cope with schizophrenia.

Individuals who are considered at risk of schizophrenia (e.g. a child of someone with the disorder) and are complaining of anxiety, depression, and/or insomnia should be treated for these complaints, be educated on addressing stress factors in their lives, and be closely monitored for development of psychosis.

MEDICATION AND SIDE EFFECTS

This subject is dealt with in detail in Chapter 8. It is worth mentioning, however, that young people who suffer a first episode of psychosis tend to be more sensitive to the effects of antipsychotic medication. An adolescent with schizophrenia should, therefore, be given a low dosage of medication to start. If it is evident that the dosage is insufficient, it should be increased very slowly. In general, young people require much lower doses in order to have their positive symptoms effectively treated. The advantage of lower dose medication is the avoidance of side effects. An initial period of approximately one week should determine if the ill person is tolerating the medication (e.g., symptoms are decreasing with minimal or no side effects). If there is no significant change in symptoms after four to six weeks, then another type of antipsychotic medication should be considered. Much of the improvement the ill person will experience will occur in the first six months of treatment.

A maintenance dosage of antipsychotic medication should be continued for at least one to two years (if not indefinitely), and be closely monitored. Psychosocial treatment should be ongoing during this time, with full access to available support services.

REINTEGRATION

One of the goals of early intervention is to facilitate the ill person's return to his/her normal activities as soon as possible. The ill person must be ready to face the challenge of returning to his/her life in the community, and thus the timing and pace of reintegration must be handled carefully (as mentioned above). Readiness will depend on the rate of recovery from positive symptoms, which could take days or weeks. The treatment team can assist by providing psychoeducation and psychosocial rehabilitation. These services will help assess the ill person's ability to maintain his/her pre-illness academic or career goals; explore the ill individual's interests and strengths to see if new activities are more suitable; examine his/her living conditions and

ability to live independently, and help the ill person make suitable living arrangements. They will also set goals for returning to social settings.

The purpose of rehabilitation is to teach the ill person how to negotiate his/her need for support within the various environments in his/her life. For example, if returning to school, the ill person may require some modifications to his/her curriculum, and/or some study aids. If returning to a job, the ill individual may need to negotiate some changes in responsibilities, or a change from full-time to part- time working hours. Financial assistance and/or disability benefits may be necessary, and the ill person needs to be educated on how to obtain them. He/She may also need help with day-to-day living skills.

The longer the ill person is removed from a near normal life-style, the more difficult it will likely be for him/her to reintegrate. It is to the ill person's advantage to receive early interventions (e.g. psychoeducation and psychosocial rehabilitation) to help him/her return to a normal (or near normal) level of functioning, and family members should strive to obtain the appropriate services for the ill person as soon as he/she is stable.

ALCOHOL/SUBSTANCE ABUSE

For people with schizophrenia, alcoholism and other substance addiction occurs up to fifty percent more often than in the general population. It is important for family members to be aware of the signs of alcohol and/or substance abuse, and to understand that the problem may be an indication of the presence of psychosis or the early stages of schizophrenia. They also need to understand the reasons why alcohol and street drugs are dangerous for people with schizophrenia. Chapter 8, section 4, provides more detailed information on this subject.

Family members are advised to pursue integrated mental health and substance abuse services for the ill person with an addiction.
Treatment should emphasize strategies to solve an existing alcohol or drug habit (e.g., professional help; self-help groups; avoiding problem environments; learning to say "no"). It should also help ill individuals to understand the advantages of abstaining from alcohol and street drugs, and use motivational techniques to promote a healthy lifestyle.

BEST INTERNATIONAL EARLY INTERVENTION PRACTICES

EPPIC (The Early Psychosis Prevention and Intervention Centre)

One of the two most prominent pioneers in best practices for early psychosis intervention is the Early Psychosis Prevention and Intervention Centre in Melbourne, Australia. It was developed by Patrick McGorry in June 1992. Created in a multicultural urban setting, the Centre is an integrated and comprehensive psychiatric service. EPPIC's goal is to serve the needs of older adolescents and young adults with emerging psychotic disorders. Through its programs, the Centre strives to reduce the extended period of delay between the first episode of psychosis and access to appropriate treatment in an appropriate environment. It provides assertive outreach to young people, some of whom are likely to have left their childhood home, and not have connections to family physicians. The bulk of the Centre's patients have already experienced a first episode of psychosis. In these cases, the Centre works to reduce the damage created by the illness (e.g., strained social and family relationships, derailed academic or vocational prospects, substance abuse, and behavioural problems). The Centre also plays an active role in educating people in the community who are likely to be involved with youth; for example, school counsellors, youth agencies, general practitioners, etc. EPPIC is also experimenting in developing interventions for the early stages of schizophrenia.

One of the goals of EPPIC was to remove the trauma and stigmatization young people experienced when they were treated in hospital settings designed for older patients with established illnesses. The clinic began as an inpatient unit, however, moved out of the Royal Park Hospital and into the Centre for Young People's Mental Health.

Since its inception, EPPIC has been successful in significantly reducing the number of admissions to hospital for acute-episode patients. It has also achieved significantly lower re-admissions and total time spent in hospital. The program has been meeting its goals of reducing treatment delays (as measured against a pre-EPPIC sample), getting ill people to adhere to their treatment plans, and successfully treating young ill people with lower doses of antipsychotic medication.

Evaluations show a twenty-five percent improvement in functioning at the twelve-month follow-up in patients cared for under the EPICC program as compared to pre-EPPIC patients.

The Centre's core services include:

• The Youth Access Team (mobile crisis assessment and treatment team)

• Outpatient case management (OCM)

• An inpatient unit

• A group program

• Cognitively-oriented psychotherapy of early psychosis (COPE)

• Family work

• PACE clinic (the Personal Assessment and Crisis Evaluation clinic), and

• Other sub-programs related to the treatment of psychosis

The Youth Access Team is a multidisciplinary mobile crisis assessment and treatment team. It is available 24 hours-a-day, seven days-a-week. YAT serves ill people experiencing a first episode of psychosis between the ages of fifteen and twenty-nine years. It provides crisis intervention in as little as an hour (for urgent referrals), in a manner that minimizes the stress to the ill individual. It will carry out assessments in an environment that is comfortable for the ill youth, such as home, school, or doctor's office. The team provides intensive treatment, making daily visits (if necessary) to establish a relationship that the young ill person trusts, and to engage him/her in treatment. This approach allows the individual to recover as quickly as possible in familiar, supportive surroundings, with minimal disruption to regular activities. YAT also offers support and information to both ill individuals and their families. As the ill person begins to stabilize, the team will introduce the ill person to the full range of services of EPPIC. YAT provides information on psychosis to professionals in the community and to the general public. The team also plays a key role in forming close links with other service providers.

If treatment in a hospital setting is necessary, the YAT staff work to minimize the trauma of hospitalization. EPPIC has an inpatient unit that is designed especially for young people experiencing a first episode. The goal of this service is to treat the ill person in a manner which reduces the disruption of a hospital stay, and to make the stay as short as possible. It is closely linked with all the other services of the Centre, and staff members help the patient to plan for transition to other programs in EPPIC. The facilities at the inpatient unit include:

•   Recreational activities (ping-pong, board games, sports equipment, art supplies, television, computers, and books)

•   Interpreting services (free-of-charge)

•   A direct line public telephone for patients to stay in contact with their families, and

•   All meals including specific dietary needs

Family and friends are encouraged to visit the patient while at the clinic, and visiting hours are supportive of this goal. A phone number for the physician and nurse assigned to each patient is made available to the families, encouraging open dialogue for the family's benefit.

Once the ill person's situation has stabilized, he/she is cared for using an outpatient case management approach (OCM). A case manager offers sound, practical advice as quickly as possible to the ill person in order to establish a good working relationship, which in turn promotes adherence to the treatment plan. The treatment plan includes psychoeducation and psychotherapy, and strives to help the ill person function in his/her various roles (e.g., at school, social events, sports activities, home, etc.). The OCM will assess the effectiveness of the ill individual's drug therapy. Crisis intervention is also available to ill young people. Cognitive therapy is available for ill people who struggle with depression, post-trauma reactions, anxiety disorders, and lowered self-esteem on an individual basis. The ill person stays under the care of the case management team for up to two years.

The role of the family in supporting a young person with schizophrenia is highlighted in the EPPIC program. Families are treated as collaborators in the treatment plan. Psychoeducation (in the form of both information sessions and family support groups), practical problem-solving, supportive psychotherapy, and family therapy services are available to family members. EPPIC strives to help families as they adjust to the illness by reducing the distress and burden of the first episode, and by teaching coping skills. It offers a four-week series of psychoeducation sessions. The program runs continuously throughout the year, providing information to family and friends on psychosis, treatment approaches, recovery, and maintenance of stability. It is complemented by a family education and support program that offers ongoing information and support to family members. The program also offers the opportunity for families to share ideas with other people in similar situations. EPPIC also provides service to individual families who want to talk about their experiences and concerns, and get help with specific problems relating to the first episode of psychosis.

EPPIC offers an extensive list of group programs to enhance its service. The table below provides a sample of the subjects encompassed by the group program.

A Group Program Worker (GPM) is assigned to each individual in order to help the ill young person identify his/her strengths; to suggest areas he/she might like to work on, and to help the person set goals and create a plan of action to meet the goals. The GPM also provides support and encouragement to the person, helping to find ways to overcome barriers to their goals, and helping the person recognize and build on existing strengths. EPPIC's group program offers recovering individuals an opportunity to: learn new skills; discover new interests; increase confidence and sense of control in life; develop personal strengths and relationships, and make plans for the future.

The PACE (Personal Assessment and Crisis Evaluation) outpatient clinic is closely associated with EPPIC and performs a research and education function. It also plays a key role in assessment, monitoring, and support for ill youth who are believed to be at imminent risk of developing psychosis, acting as a referral point to and from other agencies. PACE offers psychological and medical treatments designed to improve and enhance coping strategies. The purpose is to treat the symptoms the ill person is suffering (e.g., insomnia, depression, anxiety) in order to delay the onset of psychosis, and hopefully prevent the development of full-blown schizophrenia. Clients are monitored to help the clinic perform research of pre-psychosis symptoms. They are also examined for brain structure, neuropsychological processes, and drug and alcohol use. Treatment approaches are also evaluated to develop research for those at risk of psychosis. Participants attend PACE for approximately one year on an as-needed basis.

EPPIC is a comprehensive early intervention program, and is highly regarded as a best practice in early interventions for people with schizophrenia.

BUCKINGHAMSHIRE COUNTY, UK

The first (in chronological order) of the two most prominent pioneers in best practices for early psychosis intervention exists in a semi-rural area of England. It was developed by Ian Falloon. The project began in 1984 in a county with a population of thirty-five thousand and a well- established network of family practitioners. Its main goal was to fully integrate mental health care services with primary health care in order to facilitate early detection before a first episode of psychosis. The program is based on teamwork between family physicians and mental health teams, who train general practitioners to detect mental illness in its early stages. If early signs of a mental disorder present themselves, the mental health team assists the family physician to complete a comprehensive psychiatric assessment. Then an early intervention program including psychoeducation, stress management, and medication is designed for the ill individual.

As soon as mental illness is suspected, the ill person and his/her family are educated on the disorder, the available treatment, and the likelihood of recovery. Families involved in the program report that education at this early stage was very useful. It helped them support the ill person, and it promoted teamwork within the family unit.
Early education also meant that the ill person was informed before consenting to treatment, promoting his/her buy-in to a treatment plan. Ill

individuals and families are taught stress management skills and problem-solving techniques in their own home environment. The treatment team follows the progress of the ill person and his/her family with regular visits. If difficulties or disabilities persist, they are addressed through psychosocial rehabilitation.

Nursing care is made available to all people in their home, and is supported by an assertive outreach team that also performs crisis management. Upon the recommendation of the mental health team, the family physician prescribes small doses of neuroleptics if the ill individual shows early signs (prodromal stage) of schizophrenia (such as insomnia or concentration difficulties). The medicine is usually taken for only a brief period (e.g., a week). Both ill individuals and caregivers are trained to recognize specific prodromal symptoms, and the ill individual is regularly monitored by both his/her physician and the assertive outreach team. The hope is that the ill person achieves a rapid recovery after this brief integrated intervention.

The results of the program have been very positive. In a four-year evaluation period, only one of fifteen cases developed into full-blown schizophrenia. While the others exhibited patterns of symptoms associated with schizophrenia, they fully recovered. When compared to an early study in Buckinghamshire County, this amounted to a ten- fold reduction in the incidence of schizophrenia. While the results may

be somewhat flawed (due to people moving out of the area, and lack of controlled circumstances) the approach has proven promising for prevention of schizophrenia, and is highly regarded as a best practice in early intervention.

CONCLUSION

Adoption of the concept of early intervention is now widely accepted as a success story in the field of schizophrenia research and treatment. Programs that specialize in early intervention and prevention are making good headway into helping individuals with schizophrenia to make better and more complete recoveries. Breaking down the barriers to early intervention (recognition, acceptance, and access to appropriate treatment) is an important goal toward bettering the quality of life for individuals with schizophrenia, and their families. The more we improve public education on this subject, and the more our health care systems improve the pathway to care for our ill family members, the brighter the future will be.

CHAPTER 6: Dealing With Crisis Situations

DO'S & DON'TS

During a crisis episode, the ill person will exhibit some or all of the following symptoms: hallucinations, delusions, thought disorder, and disturbances in behaviour and emotions. Families who have been through these psychotic episodes warn that no amount of preparation can fully protect you from the shock, panic, and sickening dread you will feel when someone experiences psychosis. It is important to understand that the ill person may be as terrified as you are by what is happening: voices may be giving life-threatening commands; snakes may be crawling on the window; poisonous fumes may be filling the room. You must get medical help for the individual as quickly as possible, and this could mean hospitalization. If he/she has been receiving medical help, phone the doctor or psychiatrist for advice.

Otherwise, try to get him/her to an emergency department of a hospital or a mental health clinic. If there is a Crisis Hotline available in your community, you may also call it for help.

DO'S

- Try to remain as calm as possible

- Decrease other distractions; turn off the television, radio, etc.

- If other people are present, ask them to leave the room

- Speak one at a time

- Try saying, "let's sit down and talk," or "let's sit down and be quiet." Speak slowly and clearly in a normal voice

- Make statements about the behaviour you are observing: "I/We feel that you are afraid/angry/confused. Can you tell me/us what is making you afraid, etc." Avoid patronizing, authoritative statements such as "you are acting like a child," or "you'll do as I say, young lady"

- Repeat questions or statements when necessary, using the same words each time. Don't rephrase the question in the hope that this will make it clearer. Keep sentences short and simple

- Allow the ill person to have personal space in the room. Don't stand over him/her, or get too close

• Understand that too much emotion on your part can upset him/her further

DON'TS

• Don't shout. If the ill individual appears not to be listening to you, it may be because other voices are louder

• Don't criticize. Someone who is experiencing psychosis cannot be reasoned with at this point

• Don't challenge the ill person into acting out

• Avoid continuous eye contact

• Don't block the doorway

• Don't argue with other people about what to do

It is far better, if possible, to have the ill person go to the hospital voluntarily. If you do not think he/she will listen to you, see if a friend can talk the ill person into going. Some have found that presenting the person with a choice is more effective. "Will you go to the hospital with me, or would you prefer that John take you?" Such an approach may reduce the ill person's feeling of helplessness. Offering choice, no matter how small, provides some sense of being somewhat in control of the horrible situation in which ill persons find themselves.

Be aware that a psychotic episode may involve violence. In such situations, there is no time to talk calmly to the ill person, or to phone the doctor or psychiatrist to ask for advice. Because the individual is in an altered state of reality, he/she may try to act out the hallucination

— for example, shatter a window. Ill individuals may threaten to harm themselves, to hurt you, or to damage property. In such situations, you must do whatever is necessary to protect yourself and others (including the ill person) from physical harm. It may be that the wisest course is to leave the premises. The alternative might be to secure him/her in a room while you phone or go for help. Such an action, however, is advisable only under extreme circumstances. Also, it is probably unwise to drive the ill person to the hospital by yourself. In such charged situations, your only choices may be to phone a Crisis Hotline, or the police. Keep in mind that the police (and a crisis response team) have authority under your provincial mental health laws to take the ill person to the hospital if he/she meets the criterion of the legislation.

Crisis situations are indeed taxing on your physical and emotional strength. The more you stay in control of your reactions, the better you will be able to cope, and to help the ill person at this crucial time. Remember, this period will pass!

POLICE INVOLVEMENT

Families who have been through a crisis often found themselves hesitant to call the police. They felt that they would be treating their relative as a criminal, and that they would be giving up and abandoning the person. However, in some situations there is no other choice.

Many families discover that the statement, "I am calling the police," calms their relative. It may let the person know that his/her behaviour will not be tolerated. One father said that the sight of the police uniform helped to diffuse the situation. But another father, disagreeing with this tactic, warned that because his daughter was paranoid, seeing a police officer in her home was like waving a red flag, and infuriated her further. Try to trust your instincts: you know the ill person better than most, and have a better chance of judging how he/she may respond to different tactics.

If you phone the police, explain that the ill person is in urgent need of medical help, and that he/she has been diagnosed as having schizophrenia (if this is the case). Briefly describe what he/she is doing — making threats, damaging property – and state that you need police assistance to get him/her to a hospital. Make sure that the police know whether the ill person is armed, and whether or not there are accessible weapons in the home.

When the police arrive, be prepared for a variety of responses. Some police officers are specially trained to know how to handle psychiatric emergencies. Some police officers have little knowledge of, or experience in, dealing with this sort of crisis. Some officers may be extremely sympathetic, while others may be quite apathetic. You might be asked by the police to lay a charge. Be sure you understand the implications of this action: ask the police what they are. Know too that your own attitude or emotional state may be a factor in conditioning police reaction. In your record, document everything that happens when you phone the police: note how long it took for someone to respond to your call; note the officers' names and badge numbers; note briefly how they treated you, and how they handled the situation.

Once in your home, the police will try to assess the situation and decide what should be done. While the police are present, you may have a chance to phone the ill person's doctor or psychiatrist to ask for advice. Inform the police if you have been advised by the doctor to take the person to a particular hospital.

After the police have the information they need, they may take the ill person to a hospital emergency department. If the person refuses to go the hospital, the police have the authority under provincial mental health legislation to force him/her to go. The specific criteria the police officer uses to determine if a compulsory examination is warranted may differ from province to province. Essentially all legislation provides that if the person appears to have a mental disorder and appears to present an actual or potential danger, either to him/herself or others, then the police may enforce a visit to the hospital. It is the responsibility of the police to report all relevant information to the attending physician. They are usually required by law to stay with the ill individual until an assessment is carried out. If you have not been able to go with the police to the hospital – although you should go if at all possible — be sure to follow up with the attending police officers. We also recommend that you speak directly to the attending physician.

You may need to ask the emergency head nurse for help to reach the doctor. You also need to find out if the ill person has been admitted to the hospital, and whether or not treatment is being given. Find out the name of the admitting physician. Be sure to keep a record of all this information.

EMERGENCY PLANNING

Contributing families recommend strongly that you have an emergency plan in place for crisis episodes. For example:

• Keep a list of phone numbers handy for: the police, the doctor, the psychiatrist, and an emergency centre for psychiatric admissions. Find out if there is a Crisis Hotline in your region

• Ask the ill person's doctor or psychiatrist (ahead of time) which hospital (if necessary) to go to in case of an emergency

•	Know which family members, friends, and caregivers the ill individual might trust most in an emergency

•	Find out whom you can phone for support at any time of the day or night

•	If applicable, decide who will take care of other children

•	Consider explaining the situation ahead of time to your local police department to make them aware of your circumstances, and get their advice on emergency responses

•	Know that the crisis situation may be less frightening to the ill person if the emergency procedure has been explained and is anticipated

In crisis situations, you expect the ill individual to be admitted, if not voluntarily, then involuntarily. However, this may not be the case.
He/she may refuse to be admitted, and the medical examination may not result in an assessment that would support involuntary admission. If you are not able to be at the hospital, it is possible that the person may be allowed to leave before you are notified. If he/she is not admitted involuntarily, yet admission is recommended, families who have been through the experience strongly suggest that you consider telling your family member that returning home is not an option.
Without the alternative of returning home, the hospital may appear to be a safe haven to the ill person.

It isn't always easy to make decisions during a crisis. If you've already experienced a crisis, make plans so you will be prepared in case it

happens again.

CHAPTER 7: Acute Episodes

If ill persons have an acute flare-up of symptoms, short-term treatment strategies are needed. Whether or not they need admission to hospital, you and the treatment team will need to consider immediate safety, a full assessment, and short-term treatment measures. Once the acute phase has passed, ill individuals, family and treatment staff can consider medium and long-term treatments.

HOSPITALIZATION

When the ill person has an acute psychotic episode, hospitalization may be necessary — depending on the nature of the episode.
Sometimes, an episode is mild or moderate in severity, and does not require the security or level of observation, and intensity of
treatment, provided by a hospital. In these cases, intensive outpatient treatment can achieve all that would be accomplished by admission to hospital. When a psychotic episode is more severe, admission is likely necessary. Admission depends on various factors, including the range of alternative outpatient services, the ability of the ill person to function at home, and the availability of support from community services, friends, family, and caregivers.

It is always preferable for a person to voluntarily consent to being admitted to hospital rather than being admitted involuntarily. Voluntary admission is not possible, however, if the person is not mentally capable of consenting to the admission. Sometimes there are potential problems involving safety that preclude voluntary admission. In these cases, involuntary admission to hospital is then usually the only option. Involuntary admission criteria are set out in your provincial mental health legislation. The specifics may differ between provinces, but all mental health laws require that the person have a mental disorder, and appear to present an actual or potential danger, either to him/herself (e.g., either through harm or deterioration) or others. (See the section Legal Issues on page 171 for more information
on involuntary admission and safeguards.)
In most jurisdictions an involuntary admission to hospital can be made when one physician, after examining the ill person, issues a certificate

under the Mental Health Act. This authorizes the person's admission to hospital for a short time (e.g., one to three days) for examination and emergency treatment. A second medical certificate must be issued in hospital in order for the person to remain in hospital for longer periods. As mentioned on page 39 if the person refuses to see a physician, it may be possible for a judge to order the person to have a compulsory examination, which can lead to involuntary admission. In addition, as mentioned under the section
Police Involvement on page 85, the police may be able to force the ill person to take an examination if he/she meets the criteria specified in the provincial mental health legislation.

If the ill person is admitted to hospital, the first priority is to ensure his/her safety. To do so, hospital staff will need to know his/her medical and psychiatric history including a complete history of medication and allergic reactions. If the immediate safety of the ill person is at risk, he/she will likely be medicated promptly. For agitated or aggressive patients, short-acting medicines are sometimes needed. These can be either antipsychotics, or benzodiazepines (e.g. Valium or Ativan). It is best if the ill individual agrees to take oral medication, giving him/her
a sense of participation in resolving the crisis. If he/she cannot be convinced, however, the physician can insist on injectable medicine.

Once safety is established, a full assessment can begin. The first step is often a thorough psychiatric examination, and a psychosocial assessment regarding the ill person's entire life circumstances. Family members or close friends can provide crucial information, both about the circumstances leading up to the current episode, and about relevant personal history. A complete physical check-up, which can include blood and urine samples, is usually arranged at this stage.

When admitted to a hospital, the staff may suggest that the family take the patient's valuables and money home, or they may be kept for safekeeping until discharge. Some families suggest that it is worth making a list of these and any items of clothing and other personal effects that the ill person takes to the hospital. This can be helpful to hospital staff, and is a safeguard against subsequent misunderstandings.

The results of a full assessment should provide a diagnosis, and a preliminary treatment plan. For in-patients, that plan almost always includes daily medication. It should also include good nursing care, and emotional support provided by hospital staff. Regardless of the severity of the acute episode, hospital staff will treat the ill person as a sensible and sensitive human being. In the first few days of the acute phase of illness, it is the medication together with a therapeutic environment that makes up the bulk of treatment efforts.

Once medication and support are successful in reducing symptom severity, more insight-oriented activities can be added to the treatment plan. A number of treatment activities can be added in the later stages of hospitalization (or at home if not hospitalized) once the worst of the episode is over. To the degree that ill individuals becomes able, they can:

- learn more about the illness
- if it was a relapse, try to figure out what may have triggered it
- negotiate a more long-term treatment plan with local mental health services
- plan for a gradual return to work or school, after the leave of absence; and
- begin to resume recreational activities

Not every patient will be able to begin long-term treatment activities after a few weeks in hospital; many will need a longer stabilization phase. In the short-term, however, it is crucial that family members and caregivers build a constructive relationship with the treatment team.

For more information on rehabilitation, refer to Chapter 14, <u>Best Practices in Rehabilitation</u>.

BUILDING RELATIONS WITH HEALTH PROFESSIONALS

One of the strongest findings in the research literature is that the regular involvement of family members and caregivers has an important positive effect on the life of persons afflicted with schizophrenia. Regular involvement can begin at the assessment stage, and continue throughout the acute and long-term stages of treatment.

Below are some suggestions that can help you build a constructive relationship with hospital staff. The nature of your involvement during outpatient care will be discussed in a later section.

Your main goal during the treatment of an ill person's acute episode, whether in or out of hospital, is to establish effective communications with mental health professionals. When an ill person's family arrives at the hospital, they are in a state of panic and shock. They want to know what is going on and what will happen next. They do not understand the complicated hospital procedures. Experienced families advise that it is important to remember your objective – to get appropriate help for the ill person. They suggest a number of things you can do that will assist you in your efforts:

• Keep a record of everything while you still remember. List the questions you ask, the responses you're given, the names and phone numbers of the staff attending the ill person. Keep a record of the treatment given, including dates and times. Keep copies of anything you mail, and all notices and letters you receive from the hospital

• Recognize that hospital staff and other health care professionals are there to help the ill individual. Make it clear that you understand that this is their prime responsibility, and that you are ready to do all you can to help them. Try to establish a partnership type of relationship between the psychiatrist, the ill person, and yourself

• Find out the names of the assigned psychiatrist, psychiatric nurse, and social worker. These are the people responsible for the treatment of the ill person. You should be able to communicate with them if you have any questions or concerns

• Be polite and assertive when talking to hospital staff. Use sentences such as, "Please help me", "Please tell me where I can get information about..."

• Ask for a meeting with the assigned psychiatrist and social worker. Try to get to know them at the first meeting. Come prepared with a written list of questions. Let them know of your willingness to provide them with information about the ill person

• Keep all conversations to the point. Ask for specific information. Some sample questions to ask the health care professionals are: What specific symptoms are you most concerned about?

What do these indicate? How do you monitor them? What is the medication being given? How often? How much? Are there any side effects? What can be done about them?

• Ask for clarification if you don't understand. Do not settle for jargon and vague information

• If the psychiatrist is too busy to talk to you, write out what you want to ask or say (in point form), and deliver (or fax) the letter to his/her office

• If you phone to speak to someone who is not available, leave your name, the patient's name, and your number. Let them know the best times to call, and ask them to leave information on your voice mail/answering machine if you aren't available

• Consider having a friend or relative who is less directly involved come with you to meetings at the hospital. This person's role is to remain calm and reasonable should you become overwhelmed by emotion and frustration

• If you feel that the patient is being badly treated or is not receiving adequate care, and if polite approaches to the treatment team fails to resolve your concerns, you may wish to raise the matter with the case manager or another person in charge. If this does not resolve the problem, you should write a letter and send it to the head of the hospital, or clinic. Be specific and brief in your letters. Consider sending copies to the College of Physicians, Nursing, etc., if you think it appropriate

• Become a member of SSC. When all else fails, help from this organization may possibly allow you to cut through hospital red tape and get answers

Families who have had loved ones hospitalized warn that you should avoid actions that are not helpful:

• Do not be rude. Do not let your fears and anxieties turn into anger. Do not approach the situation with a chip on your shoulder. The illness is the enemy, not the hospital staff

• Do not bother the staff with unnecessary special requests and excessive demands

• Do not make long, detail-filled telephone calls to the staff

• Do not allow yourself to be intimidated. Do not try to intimidate the staff

• Do not come late to appointments. If your appointments are cancelled repeatedly, put your concerns in writing

Some tips on relating to the hospitalized ill person include:

• Familiarize yourself with the routines of the ward

• Discuss what is happening with the ill person. Tell him/her about

66

your efforts to help the situation

• Don't spend every day/all day, with the ill individual while he/she is in the hospital as your continual presence may interfere with the treatment process

• Respect the ill individual's wishes. If, for example, he/she seems upset by long family visits, make your visits brief and share them with other loved ones and friends

• Do not undercut staff or criticize specific staff members in front of the ill person

• Do not criticize training or activity programs in front of the ill individual

• Consider the ill person's complaints realistically. Act on those complaints that appear to be real rather than imagined

• Do all you can to make it clear to the ill person that this period of hospitalization is important for his/her health

PLANNING FOR DISCHARGE

When the ill person is in the hospital, make sure the staff is aware of your desire to be involved in discharge planning. The discharge plan should begin as soon as possible following admittance. A patient's discharge plan may involve a number of people. Overall coordination of the plan, however, should be the responsibility of one person: a designated nurse, case manager, team leader, social worker, or other caregiver (depending on the hospital's patient care system). It is important to find out who the person in charge is, and direct your communications to him/her. Families suggest that a letter to this person is often more effective than a telephone call. An example of such a letter would be:

Thank you for the care you are giving my son,

(If you can, give a specific example of help that has been particularly important to him.) I would like to meet with you to learn about and discuss options for discharge and continuing care.

Families also suggest that you have a note put on the ill individual's file to remind staff to alert you about approaching discharge. Hospitals are busy places, and the staff may forget to keep you informed.

In most provinces and territories, a social worker will be assigned to the ill person during the hospital stay. This person can advise you and the ill individual about the social services and community programs available upon discharge. He/she can also help advise whether it is best for the ill person to return home, or if alternative housing should be considered. It is important to involve family members, including brothers or sisters, in meetings with the social worker. Be sure to consult with the psychiatrist on all plans for the ill person. If the ill individual has had multiple hospital admissions because he/she does not take treatment in the community, assisted treatment mechanisms are provided by provincial mental health legislation and should be discussed with the psychiatrist. Examples of assisted treatment mechanisms include conditional leave from hospital and community treatment orders (again, these may differ from province to province). (See the section on Legal Issues on page 170 for more information.) It is important that the advice of both the social worker and the psychiatrist are in sync.

You will likely have a number of concerns about what will happen when a person with schizophrenia returns home after discharge from the hospital. You need to know how to behave towards him/her, what to say, and what expectations are realistic. Families who contributed to this book recommend that you should strive to help the ill person to become as independent as possible, consistent with the extent of the disability. The ill person's ability to do so will depend a great deal upon what he/she was like before becoming ill. The age of onset of the illness may also be a factor in how the ill person can cope.
Normally, the more skills and social development acquired before the illness, the greater the person's ability to function.

Keep in mind that you have your limitations: you may not be able to be all things to the ill person.

The process of helping the ill person achieve greater independence really starts upon discharge from the hospital. Recognize that it will involve much trial and error. Families who have been through this experience urge you to keep the process in perspective with schizophrenia as with any other major illness – heart disease, cancer, diabetes – where the ill person and the family must learn to cope with new and more demanding circumstances. For the discharged person, diet, exercise, work and social obligations will represent a considerable challenge. Taking medication regularly and attending therapy sessions may need to become part of the person's lifestyle for the first time.

Family members and friends need to learn the most effective ways of speaking to, and behaving toward, the person who is ill.

One of the first things you should do before the ill person returns home is to think about basic safety precautions. Although you may be hopeful of a permanent or long-term remission, this is not the typical experience of the majority of people who suffer from schizophrenia. If the person is disoriented, depressed, or begins to talk of suicide, you need to be aware of the potential dangers of matches, drugs, poisons, sharp objects and so on. Many people with mental disorders are heavy smokers. You should decide ahead of time what sort of house rules you want with regard to smoking. If the ill person has shown signs of aggression or violence, it may be wise to consider putting locks on some doors. You may want to lock your car and keep the keys in a safe place. Be sure the ill person understands the risks involved of driving when tired or sleepy from medication.

A Discharge Checklist can be a useful guide to ensure that the seven main areas essential to a good discharge plan are covered:

1)   Medication information should be listed on the discharge form as soon as it is known. Instructions regarding dosage, times, and any special requirements such as the need to take the drugs with food or milk, should be noted. This information usually comes from the attending doctor(s), nurse(s), or hospital pharmacist

2)   Living arrangements must be determined ahead of time. If the ill person is not going to live with his/her family, the type of residence suitable to his/her capabilities needs to be decided. Some boarding homes provide medication supervision, while

others expect clients to be responsible for their own medication. Ensure that the ill person resides in an environment where he/she will obtain the support needed to remain in the community, thus avoiding recurrent hospitalization.

3)   Follow-up community care is necessary for all people with schizophrenia. In addition to continuity of medical care, some people

may require referrals to day programs, support groups, or alcohol and drug abuse programs, along with health professionals such as dentists, eye doctors, gynecologists, etc.

4)   Most people with schizophrenia must relearn social skills and other basic life skills to realize a good recovery. All psychosocial rehabilitation options should be included on the discharge planning form.

5)   Before the ill person is discharged, it is important that he/she understands how to recognize the symptoms of schizophrenia. It may also be appropriate to educate the ill person on birth control and sexually transmitted diseases.

6)   Arrangements for transportation to therapy appointments and activity programs should be part of the discharge plan.

7)   If the ill person requires financial assistance, the treatment team should be notified in order to ensure the appropriate applications

are filed before discharge. ●

CHAPTER 8: Treatment

TREATMENT DURING THE STABILIZATION PHASE

Discharge from hospital means only that the ill person's treatment has been properly started, and that he/she can safely continue treatment as an outpatient. It does not mean that treatment is complete.

Ill persons should leave the hospital with a treatment plan that will both minimize symptoms, and maximize their quality of life. The treatment plan will almost always include taking antipsychotic medication for an extended period of time. Beyond that key element, the treatment plan for the stabilization phase should reflect ill persons' needs, as well as their wishes or preferences. Your hospital or mental health service may offer individual or group psychotherapy, life skills training, physical activities, and occupational therapy. Outpatient staff can also provide help with respect to government welfare or disability pensions, and housing support programs. Family education programs are often separate from activities that involve the ill person, and provide help on how to understand and help the ill person.

During the stabilization phase, ill individuals may still be fragile, both neurochemically and psychologically. Symptoms of moderate severity may still be present, as medications can take many weeks or even months to reduce symptoms. As such, the best treatment activities may be more basic and gentle than they need to be in the later, stable phase. It may be better to have more structured and less complex treatment activities. Complicated psychosocial treatments, such as those described in the Stable Phase section below, can begin when symptoms have lessened, and more complex cognitive functions have had time to recover.

Sometimes outpatient treatment services are grouped together into a Day Program, where patients make a commitment to a block of group

activities for several days per week. Other services allow ill individuals to pick and choose from groups, so that their activities more closely reflect their needs. Individual counselling may or may not be part of these Day

Programs.

Outpatient treatment services are very inconsistent across the country, and even non-existent in some regions. You should be able to obtain a list of outpatient services from your local hospital, the nearest Schizophrenia Society chapter, or the Canadian Mental Health Association.

YOU ARE IMPORTANT TO THE ILL PERSON'S WELL BEING

The following suggestions may help you understand how to behave around the ill individual during the early stages of treatment. Note that what works for one individual may not work for another. Ask the attending doctor(s), social worker(s), and other health professionals which strategies are best suited to helping an ill person following discharge from the hospital, or after an acute episode.
They can guide you on the matter of interacting with the ill person: whether or how hard you should push him/her to do chores, get a job, attend school, or participate in other therapeutic programs.

•   Speak with a slow-paced and low-toned voice. Use short, simple sentences to avoid confusion. If necessary, repeat statements and questions using the same words

•   Explain clearly what you are doing, and why you are doing it. For example, "I am putting your clean clothes in your closet. You can choose which clothes you want to wear today"

•   Establish a structured and regular daily routine. Be predictable.
Be consistent. Do not say you will do something and then change your mind

•   Offer praise continually. If the ill individual combs his/her hair or shaves after three days of not doing so, comment on how attractive he/she looks

•   Avoid over-stimulation. Reduce stress and tension. For example, eating meals with the family may be too overwhelming at first

•   Persuade, but never force, the ill person to take his/her medication and to keep all medical appointments

With time, the ill person may show signs of being able to handle more responsibility. Keeping in mind the above guidelines for behaviour, here are some strategies for the next steps (once the initial adjustment period is over).

- Discuss with the ill person how he/she feels about doing more things

- Begin with mastery of self-care tasks: personal hygiene, getting dressed, and eating scheduled meals

- Assign household responsibilities that are within the ill person's abilities. Watch to see if the ill person prefers to work alone or with others. For example, he/she may like to wash dishes, but prefer not to have someone beside him/her drying the dishes

- Encourage, but never push, the ill individual to be part of social gatherings if appropriate. One or two friends over for dinner may be manageable, whereas an all-day gathering of the clan – for example, a wedding – may cause undue stress and frustration

- Discuss plans with the ill person for an outing once a week. A drive and a walk in the country may be fun, whereas a trip to the city may be too noisy and tension filled. If the ill individual enjoys coffee and doughnuts, plan a break around going to the donut shop, rather than a restaurant where menu choices may be confusing

- Do not be too inquisitive. Do not always ask questions such as, "What are you thinking about? Why are you doing that?" Talk simply about local or world events: "Did you hear about the new movie starring..."

- Understand that although it may be very difficult for the ill individual to have a conversation with you, he/she may enjoy your company in other ways. Consider watching television, listening to music, or playing cards. Talk about childhood events. Some people also appreciate being read to

- Avoid constant, petty criticism. Identify the major behaviours and learn to deal with them in an honest, direct manner. For example, in many families, lack of personal hygiene is a source of great irritation. But saying things like, "Why can't you wash?" or "You smell awful," does not have a positive effect in solving the problem. It is better to present the problem as your own. "I do not like the way you smell. I have a problem with the fact that you do not shower regularly. How can we work out an agreement that you will shower daily?"

- Be forgetful. Say something like, "I forgot the milk. Can you get it please?"

- Encourage the ill person to take responsibility. For example, leave instructions about starting dinner in case you are late getting home

73

that night. And then be late

•	Try to teach the ill person how to deal with stress in a socially acceptable manner. For example, if he/she is in a public place and begin to feel panicky, they can go to a washroom until the feeling has passed

•	Remember that family members are often the only friends the ill person has. So try to be a friend; talk as a friend would. "I'd really like to see this movie. Would you come with me tonight?"

•	If you are a member of a church, encourage someone from the congregation to befriend the ill person. (Look for someone from his/her age group.)

•	Always try to put yourself in the person's shoes. Respect his/her feelings. Saying "Don't be silly. There's nothing to be afraid of", will get you nowhere. Allow the ill person to feel frightened by saying something like, "It's all right if you feel afraid. Just sit here by me for awhile"

•	Respect the person's concerns about his/her illness. Often, those who have schizophrenia ask their families not to go public – that is, not to become a public speaker or to give interviews on behalf of their support group. Although some families may feel they have a lot to offer in terms of helping others, they may decide (for the time being) to abide by the ill individual's wishes. Others, although fully sympathetic with the ill person, may decide otherwise

"…A good family environment can be a major factor in improving the chance of stabilizing the disease and preventing serious relapses."

– Dr. Ian Falloon, et al.

TREATMENT IN THE STABLE PHASE

In planning ongoing treatment for someone with schizophrenia, it is essential to have a strategy that integrates both pharmacological and psychosocial treatments. In this sense, treatment mirrors the causes of the illness itself: it is best to think of schizophrenia as a condition where excess levels of stress trigger a pre-existing vulnerability. That being the case, the ill individual will do best when treatments target both vulnerability and stress. To do that, a combination of medicine and psychosocial treatments is used. Medicine raises the vulnerability threshold, e.g., the amount of stress a person can manage before feeling distressed. Psychosocial treatments, on the other hand, allow persons to manage the kind and amount of stressors, so they don't become excessive. The psychosocial treatments, outlined below include education, family intervention, stress management, life-skills training, and case management. First, though, let's become familiar with medication issues.

MEDICATION

Medication is the cornerstone of treatment for schizophrenia. Once the acute stage of a psychotic episode has passed, most people with schizophrenia will take medicine indefinitely. This is because vulnerability to psychosis doesn't go away, even though some or all of the symptoms do. For example, without regular medication, the chance of a relapse in 2 years is 80-90%. By contrast, the 2-year relapse rate is cut in half if a person with schizophrenia does nothing except take antipsychotic medication as prescribed. Relapse rates are even further reduced by adding other treatment measures (as described in the Psychosocial Treatment section). Thus, medication has a preventive role in the long run, as well as a symptom-relief role in the short run.

First-generation medicines were introduced between 1955 and 1980. They were used to alleviate the positive symptoms (hallucinations and delusions) of schizophrenia. Second-generation medicines have been available since 1990. They work equally well on positive symptoms, and have a documented advantage in relieving negative symptoms. It remains to be seen whether the new medicines are better for cognitive symptoms, such as memory loss and concentration problems.

Clozapine – a second-generation antipsychotic – was developed to act on a variety of neurotransmitter receptors. Risperidone was developed specifically to block serotonin and dopamine receptors equally. Olanzapine and quetiapine were developed to act like clozapine. Because they are less potent at the dopamine receptor, they tend to have fewer side effects associated with the blockage of dopamine, e.g., tremor, stiff muscles, and agitation. Unfortunately, they have their own undesirable effects, such as a tendency to gain weight. This can be more of a health hazard than stiffness and tremors. There are many kinds of antipsychotic medicines in use today. Each drug has two names: the generic or chemical name (first column below), and the brand name used by the pharmaceutical company that manufactures it (second column below). The table below lists the antipsychotic medicines currently available in Canada.

Older or First generation antipsychotics

CHLORPROMAZINE	Largactil
FLUPENTHIXOL	Fluanxol
FLUPHENAZINE	Modecate
ZUCLOPENTHIXOL	Clopixol
LOXAPINE	Loxapac
HALOPERIDOL	Haldol
PIMOZIDE	Orap
TRIFLUOPERAZINE	Stelazine
METHOTRIMEPRAZINE	Nozinan

Newer or Second generation antipsychotics CLOZAPINE

OLANZAPINE	Zyprexa
RISPERIDONE	Risperdal
QUETIAPINE	Seroquel
*ZIPRASIDONE	*Zeldox

*Ziprasidone/Zeldox is currently awaiting approval from Health Canada. It is already available in the United States (known there as Geodon), and many European countries. Developed by Pfizer, Zeldox has been proven effective in treating both positive symptoms (e.g., visual and audio hallucinations; agitated behaviour) and negative symptoms (lack of motivation and social withdrawal as well as overall psychopathology) for acutely ill patients, stable patients, and those with chronic schizophrenia. The injectable form of Zeldox is a favourable option for treatment of patients with acute agitation during psychosis (including emergencies that are characterized by uncooperative and/or violent behaviour) as compared to conventional therapies that frequently result in excessive sedation and debilitating movement disorders. Zeldox has the advantage of not being associated with weight gain or cardiovascular abnormalities.

The dosage for each individual depends on a wide range of factors, including: physical differences (such as sex, weight, metabolic rate), physical health, and the severity of symptoms. There are two basic forms of administration. The most common is pills, taken by mouth. Some medicines are also available in liquid form. Oral medication requires consistent use to ensure a steady supply of medicine, every day, to the body. Some antipsychotics are available in an injectable form. A short-acting injectable drug can be used for rapid treatment, for example, when someone is extremely frightened or agitated. A longer-acting injectable form is used when an ill person can't or won't take oral medicine every day. The June 2003 issue of the American Journal of Psychiatry reported that risperidone, the first atypical antipsychotic available in long-acting injectable form, is well tolerated and effective in schizophrenia. This increases the options for people with schizophrenia that have difficulty taking medicine on a daily basis.

Most antipsychotic medicines produce substantial improvement in about two-thirds of ill people who have a psychotic episode. Of these, about half experience a full remission of symptoms. The other half experience substantial improvements, but some symptoms are still present even though they faithfully take their medicine. Unfortunately, the remaining third fail to respond to a particular medicine — in this case, the physician will try a different antipsychotic. Many ill individuals in this group will successfully respond to a subsequent medicine, even though the first one didn't work. The choice of any particular medicine is highly individualized.

Most, but not all, physicians believe that the newer drugs are the best first choice. But sometimes an ill individual will not respond to, or will lose the effectiveness of a second-generation drug. Other times, the ill individual might find the side effects of a newer medication intolerable. In this case, it is quite sensible to consider one of the older drugs.

If the ill person has failed to respond to at least two medications, after 6-12 months of good effort, your physician may suggest clozapine (Clozaril). Clozapine is currently the best choice for people with schizophrenia who have had a poor response to other medicines.

Sometimes a physician may prescribe medicine for other symptoms, such as depression or anxiety. The ill individual might also need to take

other medicines for general health problems. There are always implications of combining drugs. The prescribing doctor must be made aware of all medications, herbs, cold remedies, coffee, cigarettes, and street drugs the ill person is using.

New antipsychotic medicines continue to be developed, guided by research strategies that are increasingly complex. Unlike with older medicines, it is no longer sufficient to show simply that a new medicine is effective for the positive symptoms such as hallucinations and delusions. Pharmaceutical companies must also evaluate improvement in negative symptoms, as well as assess the cognitive effects. The safety and tolerability (e.g., side effects) of drugs are more carefully assessed than ever before. Ill people and their families are also interested in the degree to which quality of life is improved. Governments want to be assured that new medicines are cost-effective. Scientists want to know the mechanism and site of action of new medicines, in the hope that new understandings of the cause of schizophrenia will follow. Most of these issues are assessed over many years, and clinical trials now assess particular subgroups of people with schizophrenia. For example: people with severe, acute episodes; outpatients whose condition is stable but who only partially respond to their current medicine; those with and without accompanying depression; and those with little or no response to several medications. The research that guides the development of new medication is complex because our understanding of the illness is more complex.

SIDE EFFECTS OF ANTIPSYCHOTIC MEDICINE

The most common reason people stop taking medication is that they don't understand its importance. The next most significant reason is the side effects of the medicines themselves. Side effects cause different levels of discomfort, and vary from person to person. Side effects can be classified into short-term and persistent effects.

Short-term side effects appear relatively soon after starting a medication. They are highly dependent on the particular medicine and its dosage. Short-term side effects often go away by themselves after a few days of therapy. If they do not, an alternate medication may be prescribed by the attending physician. Side effects to watch for include:

• Muscle problems: stiffness, prolonged tension, or even muscle spasms

• Movement problems: shakiness or jerkiness

• Dry mouth, blurred vision, constipation, and difficulty urinating

• Drowsiness

• Lack of energy, sometimes called lethargy

• Restless legs (akathesia)

- Dizziness when sitting up or standing up quickly

- Increased appetite and weight gain

- Change in hormones, particularly those relating to sexuality and reproduction

- Decrease in libido

- Difficulty with erections, ejaculation, and reaching orgasm (if this problem persists, your physician may consider using another drug to solve it), and/or

- Loss of menstrual periods

Persistent side effects, on the other hand, are those that don't go away when the medicine is stopped. The most common of these is tardive dyskinesia (TD), the symptoms of which are involuntary muscle movements. TD most often appears in facial movements, e.g., of the mouth, tongue and lips. Sometimes it appears as jerky movements of the limbs, or other muscles. The risk of TD increases with age, and with the length of time a person has taken the TD- triggering medicine. Sometimes, persons with schizophrenia are not so much bothered by the side effects themselves, but are embarrassed by them when they are around other people. For example, they are embarrassed by involuntary movements, or don't wish to explain to others why they have less interest or energy than they used to have. In this case, support from family and friends can be invaluable.

An acute, life-threatening side effect known as neuroleptic malignant syndrome (NMS) can occur when using an antipsychotic, especially early in the treatment process, or if dosage levels are rapidly increased. It may appear when a neuroleptic (also known as antipsychotic medication) is used in combination with other drugs. Rigidity,
hyperthermia, delirium, and autonomic instability are indicators of NMS. If these symptoms appear, a physician will order all medication stopped, and will likely hospitalize the ill person in order to establish supportive treatment and a future course of therapy.

Hyperprolactinemia is a condition wherein the levels of serum prolactin in the body are elevated. The most significant result of this condition is a deficiency in estrogen or testosterone (hypogonadism). Disturbances of the menstrual cycle and an ovulatory cycle may result; fer tility may be impaired; and sexual dysfunction may be caused or exacerbated. As well, loss of estrogen makes women vulnerable to osteoporosis, cardiovascular problems, and dementia.

If this side effect occurs, prolactin levels should be monitored by the doctor, but treatment of schizophrenia should remain the priority.

The physician may combat the problem by reducing the medication dosage, by changing to a different type of antipsychotic, or by prescribing additional drug treatments. Females should be aware that decreasing serum prolactin levels in the body (to counter hyperprolactinemia) could increase chances of conception.

A common complaint about antipsychotic medication is sudden weight gain. Some antipsychotics cause more weight gain than others. Adding another medication to combat this problem may help, but this strategy is still in the experimental stage. The key to managing weight gain is having a healthy lifestyle that includes good dietary habits. For more information on this subject, please refer to Chapter 9, Medical Comorbidity of Schizophrenia, section 3 a) on Obesity.

It is important that ill individuals and their family members understand as much as possible about side effects. This knowledge can prevent many misunderstandings — for example, you will not mistake lethargy for laziness, or become frightened by tremors, and you will be able to provide valuable information to the attending physician. As a caregiver, your observations provide the treatment team with critical information, and it is important to document all you can about how the ill person is responding to the prescribed medication. For more information about side effects, you can consult your pharmacist.

Remember these general principles of drug therapy:

• Antipsychotic drugs are, for the most part, safe drugs; however, they may cause multiple side effects that can have an adverse impact on the ill person's ability and willingness to adhere to treatment

• Side effects are a cost of antipsychotic treatment that must be monitored throughout treatment

• Side effects are not constant over the course of treatment; some (for example, acute stiffness) are more likely to be short term, and others (for example, tardive dyskinesia) to be longer term

• The ill person's own perception of the severity and importance of a side effect is a crucial component of side effect evaluation

• Discuss the issue of side effects with the prescribing doctor

PSYCHOSOCIAL TREATMENTS

Following an acute episode of psychosis and diagnosis of schizophrenia, the ill person will likely need help adjusting to life with this disorder.
For individuals with schizophrenia, coping with school, a job, living independently, and even caring for themselves can rarely be achieved without psychosocial treatment (may also be referred to as psychosocial intervention). Psychosocial treatment, can consist of one-on-one counselling or training, group support, activity programs, and/or daily monitoring and communication with caregivers.

The best strategies are those that integrate medicine with psychosocial treatment. By combining psychosocial treatments with good medication practices, the ill person will reduce the need for readmission to hospital, reduce the severity of his/her symptoms, and be less distressed by remaining symptoms. Adding psychosocial treatments increases work and school functioning, improves the quality of life, and provides needed support to ill people and their families.

The effect of adding psychosocial treatment to a recovery plan is not trivial. Earlier, we said that the effect of simply taking regular medicine is to cut in half the relapse rate, e.g., 40-50% over two years. The effect of adding family-based interventions or social skills training, for example, to good medication practices is to further reduce the chance of relapse, to 25% over 2 years. There is further evidence to show that combining medicine, family-based treatments, and social skills training can reduce the relapse rates even more.

In an illness with lifelong vulnerability, the most important treatment component is a therapeutic alliance between the ill person, the treatment team, and family members. Listening to the ill person's concerns and life goals will help family members develop empathy as well as a special rapport with the ill person – two critical components of a successful treatment plan.

Persons with schizophrenia should persistently try to set goals, and realistically assess progress on a regular basis. The intensity of treatment interventions should reflect the amount of help needed to make progress towards their goals.

The most intensive interventions are those in the first year after an acute episode of psychosis. For many ill individuals, the intensity can be reduced over time. Others, however, will continue to need frequent monitoring, crisis intervention (including after-hours services), and an intense level of service on an ongoing basis.

All treatment plans should include a crisis response plan. The ill person, like most people, will get distressed from time to time. However, if that normal distress goes on too long, or becomes too severe, it may develop into an episode of psychosis. It is therefore important to learn to recognize the early warning signs of psychosis/relapse, and to respond without delay to reduce the distress. This is best accomplished if the early signs from previous episodes, and a response plan, have been identified in advance.

The treatment team can provide services that are not strictly related to treatment. For example, they can tell you how to obtain disability benefits. They can also help to arrange alternate housing if the family is feeling too burdened. They can arrange affordable recreational activities, and help set up volunteer work when a paying job would not be possible.

A minimum level of mental health services for a person with schizophrenia should include prompt access to a physician, early involvement of family members, provision of information about the illness to the ill person and his/her family, and provision of adequate housing and financial assistance. For the minority of ill individuals who relapse frequently, and whose needs strain the ability of family members and caregivers to provide support, intensive case management is often necessary.

Psychoeducation

Like most people, individuals with schizophrenia will participate more actively in a treatment plan if they have played a part in designing it, and if they understand why each of its components is important. They need to understand the basic issues about the causes of the illness, as well as the various treatment strategies for it. They do much better when they understand their own experiences in terms of the various features of the illness, and how their specific treatment plan will

reduce their symptoms and help them achieve their goals. They need to know how the illness may complicate their problem-solving abilities, how to cope with stressors, and how schizophrenia affects their plans for the future. Education can be provided on a group or individual basis; teaching packages with designed curriculum modules are available for use with groups. As with any education program, regular information sessions with interactive discussions are much more powerful than simply reading a book or attending a single lecture.

Family Involvement

Treatment guidelines now advise the inclusion of family members right from the beginning, since they are usually the primary source of support for people with schizophrenia. At the very least, this means consulting the family in the assessment process, and considering the family perspective in preparing the treatment plan. For the sake of the ill person, as well as family members themselves, it is crucial that a working alliance develop between the treatment team and the family.

Involving the family also means providing information on the cause of the illness, including a clear statement that they are not to blame for the illness. This basic information is usually presented in several sessions, and can be provided either to individual families or in a group format. Group sessions are offered by hospitals (or clinic staff), local Schizophrenia Society chapters, CMHA, or other family associations. Treatment guidelines now encourage all families to acquire a basic understanding of schizophrenia.

Where family members are able, they can also become directly involved in the treatment of the affected individual. In so doing, course and outcome are dramatically improved: relapse rates, which are cut in half by good medication practices, can be further cut in half if the family acquires appropriate information and skills related to the pursuit of good health. Family-based treatment usually includes:

• helping family members develop effective ways of coping with this difficult illness

• improvement of communication skills

• relapse prevention strategies, including the identification of early warning signs

• stress management training, and

• ways to provide support to each other during times of crisis

Other components can be added, depending on the needs of the ill person and family. A home visit often helps to build trust, and helps the clinical staff to become familiar with the ill person's circumstances. Similarly, the needs of siblings are sometimes considered as part of the treatment plan. In light of the diverse needs of families, these issues must be addressed specifically and individually.

Many controlled research studies have shown that these treatments help all kinds of families and ill people, not just those experiencing friction or frustration. As one of the best practices in schizophrenia, family involvement in treatment can now be considered the default option. That is, it should be part of the normal course of treatment, unless there is a compelling reason not to do so.

Social Skills Training

An equally powerful psychosocial treatment is social skills training. It too, can reduce relapse rates from 50% with good medication practices alone, to about 25% over two years when added to drug therapy. Social skills can range from basic skills such as making eye contact and giving compliments, to more complex issues such as making requests, giving feedback, and generally being more assertive.

Social skills training is offered for several reasons. Firstly, the source of much stress in anyone's life is interpersonal. To learn communication skills will help most people reduce stress, and in the case of people with schizophrenia will also reduce the risk of relapse. Secondly, many people with schizophrenia are still in the process of maturing when they develop the illness. They may, therefore, be awkward or quite shy, since they haven't had the opportunity to acquire the social skills that are part of normal adolescent development. Alternatively, social skills that had been acquired may have been lost due to a lengthy illness. Finally, some people with schizophrenia find complex social situations to be overwhelming. This can be a feature of the illness itself, either in the acute or the stable phase.

By learning social skills, ill individuals can engage in as little or as much social activity as is good for them at any point in time. Not only do ill people feel better about, and do better in, social relationships, they lower their stress levels and enjoy a better quality of life. Social skills training is now one of the best practices in psychosocial treatments for people with schizophrenia.

Cognitive Therapy

Cognitive therapy has been successfully used with individuals with schizophrenia who have symptoms that are at least partially resistant to antipsychotic medication. The results are a striking reduction in the severity of symptoms. A large number of studies from a number of research laboratories have found similar effects. The result is the newest addition to the collection of best practices.

Cognitive therapy was first developed for anxiety and depression. Its basic strategy is collaborative empiricism, where the ill individual and therapist generate and then test hypotheses. For example, if an ill person has a delusion of moderate intensity that a family member is poisoning his food, then a test of that hypothesis would be to ask the family to first taste the meal, or to randomly assign seating around the supper table. Cognitive therapy strategies for hallucinations might be to consider various explanations for their timing, rather than the content of the hallucination.

Case Management

Another best practice psychosocial intervention is case management for severely disabled clients. About 10% of people with schizophrenia are so severely disabled that they cannot engage in even the most basic of out-patient treatments, such as attending an outpatient clinic. For this group, the personal and social costs of not being in treatment are staggering: ongoing severe distress, isolation, poor physical health, family burnout, and high hospitalization and other emergency services costs. Most provinces and territories now provide intensive case management, often called Assertive Community Treatment (ACT, named after the first and best known program). Here, a case manager will make weekly or even daily contact, to help plan meals, organize personal hygiene, supervise medication, and arrange visits to the dentist or family doctor. The case manager can also help the client attend a Club House program, or other structured recreational activities. Case management is offered on an unlimited basis, with a 24-hour on-call capacity, and often is in place for many years.

For more details on rehabilitation programs, refer to Chapter 12, Best

Practices in Rehabilitation.

PHYSICAL ILLNESSES

People who suffer from schizophrenia are less likely to recognize, or have recognized by others, a physical illness. It is, therefore, important that the attending physician ask specific questions to uncover any ailments. People with this disorder are subject to higher incidence of suicide, smoking, caffeine ingestion, alcohol or substance abuse, self- neglect, obesity, heart disease, and diabetes – as a result they have

a higher than normal mortality rate. They should be monitored on a regular basis for cardiovascular disease, diabetes, respiratory and genitourinary problems, and conditions involving the endocrine and neurological systems. The physician or psychiatrist with primary clinical responsibility for the ill person should monitor for these and other

physical illnesses, along with psychiatric symptoms. They should also perform reassessments along with physical examinations every year. ●

CHAPTER 9: Medical Comorbidity of Schizophrenia

DEFINITION AND FACTS ABOUT COMORBIDITY

Like all people, those who have schizophrenia can experience other illnesses. However, people with schizophrenia tend to be more susceptible to particular diseases than people in the general population. The term comorbidity refers to disorders, whether medical or psychiatric, that coexist with schizophrenia. Medical comorbidity is associated with poor physical as well as mental health. For example, some people with schizophrenia have an inactive lifestyle as a result of their disorder. This in turn can lead to obesity, and obesity leads to various health problems. So, the psychiatric disorder and medical problems are interrelated.

Nearly fifty percent of individuals with schizophrenia have a related illness, whether they are being treated as inpatients or outpatients. Susceptibility to disease increases with age for everyone. On average, people with schizophrenia have a ten to fifteen year shorter life expectancy than the general population, living to approximately sixty- one years of age. The rate of death from natural causes (e.g., disease) is twice as high for people with schizophrenia. Eighty percent of deaths by natural causes are due to cardiovascular disease, respiratory disease, or cancer. More than sixty percent of deaths are smoking related.

There are five main reasons for a higher rate of natural mortality among people with schizophrenia:

• Failure by the ill person or caregivers to recognize the medical disease

• A missed medical diagnosis by a psychiatrist or physician

• Poor treatment

• Lack of insight by the ill person (e.g., refusal to acknowledge the condition or adhere to treatment), and

• An unhealthy lifestyle (especially when cigarette smoking is

87

included)

It is important that people with schizophrenia and their families learn about comorbid conditions and how to recognize their symptoms.

While medical intervention cannot always reduce some of the factors that contribute to comorbidity, awareness by ill people and their family members can help to support lifestyle adjustments, and to get treatment that can keep related illnesses under better control.

PATIENT AND FAMILY AWARENESS

There are six primary reasons that medical comorbidity in schizophrenia goes undiagnosed:

- Psychiatrists are not looking for medical comorbidities
- There is a lack of awareness among physicians of the importance of assessing for medical comorbidity
- In some cases, physicians may be unwilling or reluctant to pursue aggressive treatment on the assumption that the life of a person with schizophrenia is not valued
- Ill individuals do not report comorbid conditions
- Related illnesses are rarely mentioned in clinical treatment guidelines
- There is a lack of access to care for people with schizophrenia, and
- Comorbidity is not viewed as part of the normal scope of psychiatry

Psychiatrists specialize in mental health. Since schizophrenia is a serious and complicated disorder, psychiatrists tend to put their treatment focus on helping the ill person to recover from the mental disability it causes. Thus it is highly possible that a psychiatrist may overlook risk factors* that have a significant effect on an ill individual's health, or miss symptoms that indicate a medical disease.

In the medical field, it is not clear who is responsible for diagnosing and treating medical disorders in people with schizophrenia. A treating psychiatrist may assume that the individual with schizophrenia is healthy unless otherwise informed, or is being monitored for medical fitness by a physician. Many ill people, however, do not have a family doctor, and have difficulty getting access to one. There are shortages of physicians in various communities across Canada, and many family physicians will not take new patients. Ill individuals may, therefore, be relying upon the treating psychiatrist for overall health care. If this is the case, it is important that the psychiatrist be aware of this situation,

and understands that the patient depends on him/her to monitor for illnesses associated with schizophrenia.

It is a good idea for family members of people with schizophrenia to consult with the ill person's treating psychiatrist on a regular basis (e.g., annually, semi-annually, or as required), especially if there are no other physicians involved in their loved one's care. (Please note that if the ill person is over the age of eighteen years, the family may require a written consent of the patient before the psychiatrist will discuss the case. For more information please refer to Chapter 11, Coping with Schizophrenia, section on Confidentiality.) The family and ill person should discuss overall physical and mental health with the psychiatrist, and appropriate testing for physical and mental condition should be performed (see Chapter 5, Early Intervention, section on What to Look for in Assessments). Complete psychological and physical assessments should provide information that will give the ill individual and his/her family as clear a picture as possible on the status of the illness, as well as overall medical health. It is essential that any existing medical problems be fully investigated. They cannot only pose a serious medical risk to the ill person (e.g., heart disease), but they could also contribute to more severe psychoses, leading to depression and a greater likelihood of attempts at suicide. Many health problems can be treated (e.g., diabetes, obesity) either with medicines or adjustments in diet or lifestyle. The sooner a problem is detected, the more likely it can be controlled, and then the risk the concern poses to the health of the ill person is decreased.

In this book, the importance of family involvement with the treatment team is emphasized. Families and caregivers help the person with schizophrenia in the management of, and recovery from, schizophrenia. Family involvement is also important to the medical health of the ill individual. The ill person may not report symptoms of conditions such as diabetes to the treating psychiatrist or physician. People with schizophrenia often lack the insight or awareness of their medical condition. They may also have trouble communicating their symptoms, or may provide incorrect medical history to the treatment team.

Individuals with schizophrenia may also be victims of a fragmented healthcare system. They may discuss their physical complaints with a nurse or case manager, but the message may not get the attention of the treating psychiatrist. It is important that families of people with schizophrenia become aware of the important medical comorbidities in schizophrenia, and familiarize themselves with typical symptoms of these conditions. Families must also ensure that either the ill person or a family member communicates accurate medical history to the treating psychiatrist, as well as any concerns or symptoms that develop.

Family members should educate themselves about the **illnesses related to schizophrenia, so they can recognize their presence in the ill person, and help the ill person get treatment.**

COMMON COMORBID CONDITIONS

The most common threats to the health of a person with schizophrenia are:

- Obesity
- Heart disease
- Diabetes

OBESITY

Obesity is both a medical comorbidity and a risk factor for other disorders. It is generally defined by a body mass index (BMI) calculation. This is a standard measurement that compares body weight to body height to determine a body mass. The Canadian Standard BMI says that a calculation of greater than twenty-five indicates overweight, and thirty and over indicates obesity.

In Canada, twelve percent of the general population is considered obese, whereas forty-two percent of people with schizophrenia are obese. Nearly half of all individuals with schizophrenia, therefore, are significantly overweight.

When physicians want to get an indication of the risk of disease from

obesity, they will often use the BMI along with the patient's waist measurement. For example, if a man's waist is less than 40 inches but his BMI is thirty-five or greater, his risk of disease associated with obesity is very high. If a woman's waist is greater than thirty-five inches and her BMI is thirty or greater, she too has a high risk of health problems. Waist measurement is important because a high waist-to-hip ratio is positively associated with heart attack, stroke, glucose intolerance, insulin resistance, and dyslipidemia (also known as the metabolic syndrome – see section on cardiovascular disease for definitions). The chart below gives you an idea of whether or not you or your family member may
be at risk of disease associated with obesity.

BMI and Risk of Associated Disease

Obesity can have serious consequences (both medical and non- medical), and can lead to the disorders and risks listed below.

Medical disorders:

- Hypertension
- Dyslipidemia
- Atherosclerosis
- Diabetes
- Gallstones
- Congestive heart failure
- Stroke
- Osteoarthritis
- Cancer (endometrial, breast, colon)

Non-medical risks for obese people with schizophrenia include:

- Not adhering to the treatment plan (including antipsychotic medication)
- Having a diminished quality of life
- Social withdrawal, and

- Stigmatization

People with schizophrenia who are also obese are three times more likely not to adhere to treatment than ill people of normal weight. It is, therefore, essential that the antipsychotic medication used by ill individuals maximize their overall quality of life, otherwise they are less likely to take the medication as prescribed, and therefore more likely to suffer from relapse. (See Chapter 8, Treatment, sections on Treatment in the Stable Phase, Side Effects of Antipsychotic Medicine, and Chapter 11 Coping With Schizophrenia, section on Encouraging Medication.)

There is a stigma that goes along with obesity. People with excessive weight tend not to be well embraced by society, and are very self-conscious as a result. This leads to social withdrawal and a diminished quality of life for many people who suffer from obesity. For people with schizophrenia, the stigma already attached to the illness, coupled with the lack of self-confidence that comes from being overweight, can seriously impact their quality of life.

Social isolation in turn can lead to increased inactivity, especially when coupled with low socio-economic status. The less active a person is, the more prone he/she is to gaining weight.

Causes of Weight Gain

Typical causes of weight gain include:
- Poor dietary habits
- Lack of exercise
- Age
- Gender
- Substance abuse, and
- Antipsychotics and other psychotropic medications

POOR DIETARY HABITS:

- Eating on the run and snacking (especially in the evening) are big contributors to an unbalanced and unhealthy diet. This problem is made worse if the snack foods are empty calorie foods (foods that do not provide good nutrients and energy for the body)

- Eating lots of fatty and sugary foods like biscuits, sweets, cakes, muffins, and chips can lead to fluctuations in blood sugar. These can give you mood swings or make you feel tired, irritable, or depressed. The same can happen if you regularly skip meals

- Eating too many simple carbohydrates produces a high sugar level in the body, which turns into fat. Simple carbohydrates include breads, starches (potatoes, rice, etc.), fruit juices, cereals

- Not eating three healthy meals a day, with a proper daily balance of protein, grains, vegetables, and fruit will likely lead to snacking, and eating inappropriate foods. Not taking the time to plan and eat a well balanced diet will likely lead to forming the poor dietary habits listed above

Lack of Exercise

Health and fitness go hand in hand. If you are fit, you will be in better condition to face life, both mentally and physically. By contrast, if we do not look after ourselves – both our physical and mental health – we will likely suffer physical health problems that can also affect our mental and emotional well being.

People with schizophrenia are particularly prone to physical inactivity. Feelings of fatigue, depression, or anxiety can drain one's energy, making it difficult to be motivated to exercise. The problem is, however, that the more inactive one is, the more tired and less vibrant a person tends to feel.

Age

As people get older, there is a tendency to want to slow down, or not feel as strong or able to be physically active. Again, the problem is that the more inactive the body is, the more likely it is to feel stiff, sore, or tired. Physical movement is necessary to maintain good blood circulation to all the body's hundreds of parts. Poor circulation, and lack of use of muscles, leads to stiffness and soreness. While activities may have to be modified as one ages (e.g., a fast paced walk as opposed to running), it is just as important to exercise when you are older.

It is interesting to note that drug-induced weight gain (see section on medications below) is lower for people over sixty years of age than for younger adults.

Gender

There is some scientific evidence that suggests females who experience schizophrenia may have a higher risk of weight gain than males. For example, research led by Dr. Tony Cohn of the Centre for Addiction and Mental Health in Toronto shows that the prevalence of obesity for women with schizophrenia is three times that of the general population. Males with schizophrenia tend to be two times more obese than men without the disorder.

Substance Abuse

For people with schizophrenia, alcoholism and other substance addiction occurs up to fifty percent more often than in the general population. Long-term alcohol abuse can lead to poor dietary habits, lack of physical activity, depression, and overall poor physical and mental condition. Alcohol is high in calories, and excessive intake means that the person is adding many empty calories (likely on a daily basis) to his/her diet. Since they are not likely to burn these extra calories off with vigorous exercise, people with schizophrenia that regularly abuse alcohol are prone to weight gain. (For more information on the impact of drugs and alcohol on a person with schizophrenia, please refer to Chapter 10, Living with Schizophrenia, section 4 on Drugs & Alcohol, and Chapter 17 Research: The Hope for a Cure, section 2 (iii) on Alcohol/Drugs Recovery.)

Antipsychotics and Other Psychotropic Medications

Many people with schizophrenia find it difficult to maintain a healthy body weight. This may in part be due to their medication, which can, in some individuals, lead to an increase in appetite. Some drugs are more likely to cause weight gain than others, so if you are bothered by excess weight, it is worth your while to discuss the matter with your physician.

All antipsychotic medications that are currently available in Canada have the potential to cause weight gain. Atypical antipsychotics may cause more severe weight gain than first-generation antipsychotic drugs. The amount and rate of drug-induced weight gain depends upon the atypical antipsychotic being used. Weight gain can plateau after a certain period of treatment (e.g., in the first few months, or not for a year).

Most weight gains are in the first year of treatment, but may continue at a slower rate for several years. Weight gains caused by drug therapy range from minimal to moderate to intermediate. Of all the atypical antipsychotic drugs, ziprasidone (not yet available in Canada at the time of writing) appears to have a neutral effect on weight gain.

The weight gain caused by antipsychotic treatment is a concern because of the significant morbidity and mortality associated with it. It also creates concern because obese individuals with schizophrenia are
thirteen times more likely to request discontinuation of their medication because of weight gain.

While the exact cause of drug-induced weight gain is not clear, it appears the physiological impact of the atypical antipsychotics leads to appetite stimulation. Ill individuals tend to increase their caloric intake (with or without changing the composition of their diet) while taking these medications.

One of the side effects of some antipsychotics can be sedation, increasing the likelihood that individuals will be less active, and therefore gain weight more easily. Some people with schizophrenia are treated with other psychotropic medications, or medications used to assist the effectiveness of antipsychotics. Some of these medications are known to promote weight gain (e.g., lithium, mood stabilizers including valproate, tricyclic antidepressants and SSRI's, and mirtazapine). Also, a drug treatment plan that combines atypical antipsychotics with mood stabilizers may result in significant weight gain. For example, a combination of lithium or valproate with risperidone is reported to cause twice as much weight gain (than risperidone alone). When these mood stabilizers are combined with olanzapine, they may create three times as much weight gain (than therapy with olanzapine alone).

When a psychiatrist or physician prescribes an atypical antipsychotic medication to alleviate the symptoms of schizophrenia, he/she should take the following factors into consideration:

- The ill person's overall health and condition
- The severity of the symptoms
- The ill person's age
- The ill individual's family history of obesity-related risk factors

•   The history of adherence to the treatment plan

•   The ill person's weight; BMI, and his/her glucose and lipid levels before medication

•   Any prior sensitivity to drug-induced weight gain

•   The ill person's tolerance level for weight gain – both from a psychological, and an overall physical health standpoint, and

•   The ill person's ability and willingness to manage an increase in his/her weight

It is a good idea for family members to meet with the prescribing physician to discuss the choice of antipsychotic treatment. You may be able to give the doctor very useful information on the ill person's background, lifestyle, condition (since the onset of illness), and family history. You can also help evaluate whether or not the ill person will likely be able to deal with the psychological aspects of a weight gain. You may also discuss ideas on how to help the ill person with a good diet and exercise routine.

Strategies to Monitor, Prevent, and Manage Obesity

•   Monitor your weight – weigh yourself weekly

•   Eat a healthy balanced diet

•   Exercise regularly (at least 3 times per week)

•   If necessary, seek help from a support group and/or health professional

•   Keep alcohol intake to a minimum, and avoid the use of street drugs; and

•   Consult with the prescribing physician at least every six to twelve months to ensure your antipsychotic treatment is maximizing your quality of life

Watching your weight makes good sense for various reasons, the most significant of which is the prevention of disease. It is also a good idea to maintain a healthy weight for your self-esteem. Maintaining your self-esteem can be closely connected with your appearance.
Gaining weight can have an adverse effect on how you feel about yourself (and thus your outlook on life in general), and may diminish your confidence in social situations.

The best way to start monitoring your weight is firstly, to get weighed. The next step is to find out whether your weight is within the healthy range for your height (ask your general practitioner, or a member of

your treatment team for guidance about what a healthy weight would be for you). It is a good idea to weigh yourself once a week if possible. Weigh yourself at the same time of day (e.g., when you first rise for the day, before lunch, before bed, etc.). This is important because your weight will fluctuate during the day.

Another good way to monitor your weight is to keep a check on whether your clothes fit you – if they start to become tight, it is a sign that you are gaining weight.

Of course the key component to maintaining a healthy weight is to eat a healthy balanced diet. To find out whether your diet is appropriate, start by keeping a food diary: make a note of your typical day's diet. For the first few days, observe what it is you eat during the day. Be honest with yourself – this exercise will help you identify potential pitfalls and problem foods, or particularly difficult times of day. At the end of the week, analyze your overall diet and try to identify your problem areas. Then, try to follow a healthy balanced diet, one that includes protein, vegetables, fruit, and whole grains. Ask a member

of your treatment team or other health professional for nutrition counselling. A nutritionist should be able to give you the types and portions of food you should be eating on a daily basis. A sensible eating plan is one that will fit in with your lifestyle so that you follow it. You should strive to eat three regular meals a day (don't skip meals), and avoid eating on the run and snacking. Planning your day's diet when you get up in the morning will help to ensure you eat well throughout the day. It is also important to avoid eating fatty and sugary foods (e.g., biscuits, sweets, cakes, muffins, and chips), and excessive amounts of simple carbohydrates (e.g., breads, starches {potatoes, rice, etc.}, fruit juices, and cereals).

If you find you need to lose weight, and find it difficult to do it alone, think about joining Weight Watchers' or a similar support type group that is designed to give you regular encouragement and help with your diet. Always consult your physician before joining such an organization.

One way to improve health and maintain a healthy weight is to exercise regularly (at least three times per week). This may be one of the last things the ill person feels like doing, especially if he/she is experiencing fatigue, depression, or anxiety. Family members are advised to encourage the ill person to exercise, perhaps by incorporating it into the family's routine. It may be helpful to note that exercise can actually make one feel more energetic, more relaxed, and improve the spirits. It is good for the mind as well as the body. It can also be a natural way to meet people. Of course it is always wise to speak to the ill individual's physician before embarking on a new exercise program, especially if the person is not used to exercising.

The ill person may wish to consult the treatment team on the subject, and get their feedback. They may have helpful tips on how to approach exercise and get fit safely.

It is quite easy to introduce physical activity into one's lifestyle. It is not necessary to join an expensive club or gym. Simply find something the ill person (or entire family) enjoys doing and set some time aside for it every week. A person is more likely to stick to an exercise routine if it is an activity he/she likes. Here are some suggestions for the ill person (or the whole family):

• If you like walking, this is an excellent form of exercise and can be done in the town or country. Set aside at least 20 to 30 minutes of the day for a walk. You could combine it with a visit to the store, or to your local day centre or community centre. Perhaps there is someone in your family or at your support group who could accompany you?

• Running groups and clubs are quite popular in urban centres. They teach you how to run, helping you to slowly build up your stamina through a pre-designed program. They meet on a regular basis (e.g., weekly) to do group training

• If there is a municipal swimming pool nearby, try swimming two or three times per week. In the winter, arenas usually offer public skating at very reasonable prices

• If you like cycling and have (or can borrow) a bicycle, find a safe route to go cycling

• Do a few more things around the home or garden. For example, household activities such as cleaning or gardening can be good exercise, and may also help you get into a good daily routine

The primary reason for avoiding the use of alcohol and/or street drugs is the serious health risk they pose to the person with schizophrenia.

In addition, alcohol adds lots of calories to a daily diet, but not lots of nutrients. If you have a regular habit of drinking alcohol, beware of the calories you are taking in. Reducing alcohol intake, or avoiding it altogether, is a positive step toward maintaining a healthy weight. It is not wise to use street drugs for health reasons, but also because they may stimulate appetite, and impair your judgment.

If the ill individual feels that the medication is the reason for his/her weight gain, and the weight gain is not manageable and is adversely affecting his/her quality of life, then a discussion with the prescribing physician about the antipsychotic treatment is warranted. The physician may change the dosage of the medication, or suggest another choice of drug treatment, or consider additional medication to help with weight management. However, the physician may first wish to do a risk-benefit analysis of the current medication. In other words, the doctor will weigh the risks and benefits of continuing the current treatment by comparing the side effects of the medication (e.g., weight gain) with the effects of psychotic episodes. One of the physician's key concerns is preventing the ill person from relapsing, but he/she will also be keeping in mind the ultimate goal of improving the quality of life of the ill individual. The physician will also be aware that patients are more likely to be motivated to continue taking antipsychotic medication if they experience more positive effects (than negative side effects) of the treatment.

CARDIOVASCULAR DISEASE (CVD)

The term cardiovascular disease refers to strokes, and diseases and injuries of the cardiovascular system which is made up of the heart, the blood vessels of the heart, and the veins and arteries throughout the body and brain. One in four Canadians is estimated to have some form of heart disease or is at risk of having a stroke. More Canadians die from cardiovascular disease than any other disease: thirty-five percent of all male deaths in 1999 were from CVD, and thirty-seven percent of all female deaths resulted from CVD.

Risk Factors for CVD

The risk of heart disease or stroke is even greater for people with schizophrenia than for people in the general population. Heart patients with schizophrenia under the age of sixty-five years who undergo cardiovascular procedures are eighty-six percent more likely to die following the medical procedure. There are two categories of risk factors for heart disease – one category is factors that can be modified, and the second category consists of risk factors that are not changeable.

Risk Factors for Heart Disease

Modifiable

- Obesity
- Diabetes
- Smoking
- Dyslipidemia
- Hypertension
- Atherosclerosis
- Psychological factors

Non-modifiable

- Advancing age
- Gender
- Family history
- Medical history
- Medication

Obesity and diabetes are not only comorbid conditions of schizophrenia, but they are also important contributing risk factors to heart disease.

Smoking is probably the most common risk factor for heart disease.

Dyslipidemia (an abnormal amount of fatty acid) is a metabolic abnormality that causes injury to the arterial walls creating problems in how cholesterol is processed in the body.

Hypertension produces structural changes within arteries that narrow the arterial openings, which may lead to aneurysms (an excessive localized enlargement of an artery) and necrosis (the death of tissue caused by disease or injury). The effects of hypertension manifest themselves after several years, and are made worse by other risk factors such as dyslipidemia, smoking, diabetes, obesity, an inactive lifestyle, high amounts of salt in the diet, and stress. Hypertension tends to increase with age.

Artherosclerosis is a form of arteriosclerosis (thickening of the walls of the arteries; also known as hardening of the arteries), and is caused by the build-up of fatty deposits.

Examples of psychological factors that contribute to heart disease include stress, anxiety, depression, and hostility.

Medical science also looks at risk factors in terms of metabolic syndrome. Metabolic syndrome occurs when three of the following risk factors are present at the same time: abdominal obesity (for men, a waist measurement greater than forty inches, and for women a waist measurement greater than thirty-five inches); a high level of fatty acids; low HDL cholesterol; high blood pressure, and high fasting glucose. People with metabolic syndrome have a significantly increased risk of diabetes and coronary heart disease. There is a chart known as the Framingham chart that doctors can use to calculate a person's ten-year risk for heart disease. The chart assesses risk based on the following risk factors: age, gender, systolic blood pressure, HDL cholesterol, smoking, and total cholesterol. A point system is used to evaluate each risk factor, and the total number of points then corresponds to a person's percentage chance of having heart disease within the next ten years.

CVD and Antipsychotics

People with schizophrenia are vulnerable to CVD, and atypical antipsychotic drugs have the potential to worsen CVD risk factors. Some antipsychotics may cause side effects such as dyslipidemia or hypertriglycemia (high lipid levels), an increase in triglyceride levels, weight gain, sedation (leading to inactivity and obesity), hyperglycemia, diabetes, sudden death from electrical problems with the heart, and complications with hypertension. The choice of antipsychotic medication must be carefully weighed against the risk of CVD.

Strategies to detect CVD risk factors:

- Get your blood pressure measured at every medical check-up
- Monitor your weight
- Get checked for metabolic syndrome
- Have your lipid levels measured, and
- Have your blood sugars tested for hyperglycemia and diabetes

It is important to have a complete check up with all of the above measurements before you begin antipsychotic treatment, and on a regular basis once you are undergoing drug therapy. (See Chapter 4, section on Initial Assessment, page 42, and Chapter 5, section on Early Intervention Strategies – What to Look for in Assessments, page 55 for more information.) If you are diagnosed with dyslipidemia, hypertension, or diabetes the physician will likely recommend medication to control these conditions.

The best way to minimize your risk for cardiovascular disease is to:

- Eat a healthy diet
- Keep active and exercise regularly
- Don't smoke, and
- Have your antipsychotic medication assessed on a regular basis (e.g., every six months to one year)

Warning Signs of Heart Problems

People with schizophrenia and their family members should be aware of the warning signs of heart trouble. They include:

- Light-headedness; dizziness
- Palpitations
- Inability to speak or make sounds
- Temporary loss of consciousness
- Difficulty breathing
- Sudden discomfort or pain that does not go away with rest
- Pain in the chest, neck, jaw, shoulder, arms, or back
- Burning pain
- Squeezing, heaviness, tightness, or pressure
- Vague pain (for women)
- Indigestion
- Vomiting
- Cool, clammy skin, and/or
- Anxiety

The symptoms can range in severity from mild to severe. If the ill person is experiencing some of the serious symptoms that may indicate a cardiac event, call 911 or your local emergency number. The person may need to be taken immediately to the emergency ward of a hospital, or be attended by a medical emergency service unit. The ill person should stop all activity and sit or lie down in a comfortable position. If he/she is experiencing chest pain, they may chew and swallow one adult 325 mg tablet of aspirin (or two 80 mg tablets). No other pain medication (e.g., acetaminophen or ibuprofen) should be taken.

If the ill person is not breathing normally, or coughing, or moving then he/she requires help from the nearest people around them. CPR (cardiopulmonary resuscitation) should be started right away, and continued until emergency help can take over. Early intervention in the case of heart attack can significantly improve the chance of survival for the ill person.

It is particularly important that people with schizophrenia pay attention to the risk factors of cardiovascular disease. Maintaining a healthy lifestyle is the best prevention against heart problems. People with schizophrenia should have regular medical check-ups to monitor for CVD risk factors.

Rare Side Effects

People with schizophrenia and their families may come across information on antipsychotic drugs that at first glance could be alarming. The Canadian Government (Health Canada) has made rulings that require some pharmaceutical companies to post warnings on their products to alert users to specific conditions or side effects that
may occur during treatment. These rulings resulted from concerns relating to a history of cardiac problems with older antipsychotics, antihistamines and sertindole. The labels do not mean that patients will experience the condition, but rather that users should be educated about the potential side effects so as to recognize signs of onset, and/or to ensure they are regularly monitored by a physician. It is also possible to have a warning that pertains to particular patient populations (e.g., those of various ethnic origins) for which there may be potential side effects. One of these potential side effects is QTc prolongation.

Prolongation of the QTc interval is a condition that may be induced by drugs such as diuretics, quinolone antibiotics, and antipsychotics. The QTc interval is the length of time that it takes for the heart ventricles to electrically discharge and recharge. An electrocardiogram can be performed on a person to measure QTc interval, and test for prolongation. For women at rest their QTc count is typically less than four hundred and fifty, and for men it is four hundred and thirty. Some drugs can cause the QTc interval to increase. A clinically significant prolongation of the QTc interval would be an increase greater than a count of thirty. If the QTc interval is increased to greater than a count of five hundred, the person may be at risk of sudden death from arrhythmia (an irregular heart rhythm or ventricular fibrillation), or a condition known as torsade de pointes. Torsade de pointes is extremely rare and unpredictable, and can lead to sudden cardiac death. Most cases of torsade de pointes have occurred in patients with a QTc interval greater than a count of five hundred on an electrocardiogram. The greater the QTc prolongation, the greater is the risk of torsade de pointes.

People with schizophrenia who have been diagnosed with a QTc interval prolongation should immediately contact a physician, and be referred to a cardiologist on an urgent basis, if the following symptoms occur:

- Light-headedness
- Dizziness
- Palpitations
- Fall in blood pressure
- Temporary loss of consciousness due to a fall in blood pressure

The physician will likely obtain an electrocardiogram, check the ill person for levels of serum potassium, magnesium, and calcium, and check thyroid hormones. He/She will also inquire about family history of loss of consciousness due to a fall in blood pressure, and any sudden deaths in the family. It may, therefore, be useful to have a family member attend the medical visit with the ill person. If the QTc interval is greater than a count of five hundred, it is a signal to the physician to change the antipsychotic treatment.

It should be noted that some people naturally have a longer QTc interval than others. Some of the contributing factors to this prolongation include:

- Female gender;
- Elderly in age;
- Electrolyte imbalance;

- Congenital long QT syndrome;

- Cardiac disease (heart attack, congestive heart failure, arrhythmias);

- Endocrine or metabolic disorders (e.g., diabetes, obesity, hypothyroidism, pituitary insufficiency);

- Central nervous system disorders (e.g., stroke, infection, trauma), and

- Drug-induced QTc interval prolongation.

Recent clinical trial studies performed on haloperidol and newer generation antipsychotics such as risperidone, olanzapine, quetiapine, and ziprasidone found modest changes in QTc intervals (that is prolongation by a count of five to fifteen) when maximum drug doses were used. It is the older antipsychotics (including phenothiazine and butyrophenones) in particular, however, that are associated with a prolonged QTc interval and torsade de pointes. Some are more prone to induce QTc prolongation than others, namely thioridazine, mesoridazine, pimozide, and droperidol.

It should be noted that QTc interval prolongation can be reversed if drug therapy is discontinued.

Individuals taking medication should understand their family history, their own medical history, and the potential side effects of the treatment they are undergoing. People with schizophrenia and their family members can ask questions of the prescribing physician, pharmacist, and other members of the treatment team to educate themselves about the antipsychotic therapy they are receiving. It is important to remember that antipsychotic treatment is a key to the recovery of the ill person.

DIABETES

Diabetes is a chronic disease that has no cure. It is a leading cause of death by disease. If left untreated or unmanaged, the high levels of blood sugar associated with diabetes can result in complications including: heart disease (which is two to four times more common in people with diabetes); adult blindness; serious kidney disease, limb amputations, and sexual dysfunction. People with schizophrenia have a two to four times higher risk of developing Type 2 diabetes than people in the general population. Type 2 diabetes occurs when the pancreas does not produce enough insulin, or when the body does not use the insulin that is produced effectively. Ninety percent of people with diabetes have this type. The risk factors associated with diabetes include: obesity (body mass index over thirty); age; a family history of diabetes; an experience with diabetes during a pregnancy; being a member of a high-risk group such as Aboriginals, Hispanics, and Africans; having a high level of cholesterol or other fats in the blood; having a more than normal level of blood glucose, and having high blood pressure or heart disease. Obesity is strongly correlated with a higher risk of diabetes. There is also some evidence that both conventional and atypical antipsychotics may cause glucose intolerance (hyperglycemia) leading to diabetes.

It is not presently clear which specific drugs have a higher or lower potential to induce diabetes. However, a 1999 study in the United States, which analyzed almost thirty-nine thousand outpatients with schizophrenia over a four-month period, found that all patients on antipsychotics had a higher prevalence of diabetes, and people on atypical antipsychotics were nine percent more likely to have diabetes than those undergoing typical antipsychotic treatment. The findings indicated that the patients completely recovered from diabetes when the antipsychotic treatment was discontinued, and that hyperglycemia promptly recurred when the antipsychotic treatment was reinstituted. This finding indicates that this side effect is reversible and drug-related. It is not yet known whether the drugs cause the diabetes or simply hasten its onset.

In a separate U.S. trial, forty-eight patients tested showed significant hyperglycemia and diabetic complications can occur during treatment with atypical antipsychotics with or without a change in weight.
Studies in the United Kingdom indicate patients taking olanzapine had the greatest risk of diabetes, and patients on risperidone or typical neuroleptics had a slightly increased risk of diabetes. In a fifty-two week controlled trial that compared risperidone with ziprasidone, two cases of diabetes were found in people on risperidone, while none were found in people taking ziprasidone. It is important to note that studies are ongoing, and conclusive evidence has not yet been established. It is also important to remember that when other risk factors of comorbid conditions of schizophrenia are considered (e.g., obesity, inactive lifestyle, etc.), the risk of diabetes is already considerably high.

Symptoms of Diabetes

People with schizophrenia and their family members should be aware of the physical symptoms of diabetes. All observations should be reported immediately to the ill individual's physician or psychiatrist.

People with schizophrenia who are over the age of forty-five years should be screened every three years for diabetes even if they do not have any other risk factors. If other risk factors do exist, they should be screened more often (e.g., every year). It is important to remember that ill people often lack the insight to recognize or complain of the physical symptoms of diabetes. Also, people with Type 2 diabetes may not display any symptoms.

Typical signs and symptoms of diabetes include the following:

- Unusual thirst
- Frequent urination
- Unusual weight loss
- Extreme fatigue or lack of energy
- Blurred vision
- Frequent or recurring infections
- Cuts and bruises that are slow to heal, and
- Tingling or numbness in hands or feet

Treatment of Diabetes

Scientists believe that lifestyle is closely linked to diabetes, and that people can prevent or delay the disease through healthy eating, weight control, exercise, and good stress management. The earlier diabetes is diagnosed, the better. Type 2 diabetes is controlled through exercise and meal planning, and may require medication and/or insulin to assist the body in making or using insulin more effectively.

The first step in treating this disease is to become educated about the condition. Knowledge is key to making healthy lifestyle choices that will keep diabetes under control. The second step is self-discipline which is essential to regulate eating habits and plan meals on a daily basis. What you eat, when you eat, and how much you eat plays an

important role in regulating how well the body manages blood sugar levels. It is particularly important that the person with diabetes maintain a healthy weight in order to control type 2 diabetes. As well, regular exercise helps to lower blood sugars in the body. Stress reduction is also important in the day-to-day management of diabetes.

People with schizophrenia who are diagnosed with diabetes may need extra help and support to adjust to the disease, and to adopt a lifestyle that helps keep diabetes under control. The treatment team may be able to help the ill individual with a diet plan, or recommend a dietitian who can help. It is a good idea for the ill individual and family members to sit down with the dietitian and discuss the lifestyle, favourite foods, and culture of the person with schizophrenia. This will help the dietitian to fit meal planning as close to lifestyle as possible, and include the foods the person enjoys eating.

DIET TIPS

•   Eat three regular meals a day (no more than six hours apart) to help your body control blood glucose levels

•   Limit foods that are high in sugar (sweets, soft-drinks, desserts, candy, jam, and honey)

•   Limit high fat foods (chips, fried foods, pastries) in order to help maintain a healthy weight

•   Eat more high fibre foods to help keep blood glucose and cholesterol levels down

•   Drink at least 6-8 glasses of water every day

•   Monitor your salt intake as high blood pressure is a potential complication of diabetes, and

•   Avoid alcohol

Healthy eating and exercise are key to controlling diabetes. It is also important to take care of your feet. High glucose levels may eventually lead to poor blood flow and loss of feeling which can lead to foot problems. In order to prevent problems with your feet, you should follow the advice below:

•   Keep your blood glucose levels in your target range

•   Wash feet daily with warm (not hot) water and pat dry

•   Check feet daily for sores, blisters, injuries, red and warm areas that change in colour, as well as any strange odour

•   Make sure to wear shoes with good support, and socks that fit well so as not to hurt your feet

- Don't walk barefoot

- Keep toenails properly trimmed; and

- Use lotion on the soles of the feet to prevent dryness and cracking

Blood Glucose Levels

As with schizophrenia, it is important for people with diabetes to take any medication that is prescribed. People with diabetes should make regular visits to their physician to monitor their condition. The physician will tell them about their appropriate target range for their blood glucose level. Everyone's target range is different. The physician will also tell the ill person how often to check blood glucose levels.

The ill person and family members must be fully trained in how to test blood glucose levels. A pharmacist or a trained health professional can tell you which blood glucose meter to purchase. You should also know:

- The size of the drop of blood needed

- The type of blood glucose strips to use

- How to clean the meter

- How to check if the meter is accurate, and

- How to code your meter

It is very important for the ill person to keep his/her blood glucose level as close to his/her personal target range as possible. The way to do this is by having good regular eating habits, an active lifestyle, and possibly taking medication. If your blood glucose level is low, it may mean that you have had more activity than usual; haven't eaten on time; eaten less than you should have; taken too much medication, or are experiencing effects of drinking alcohol.

Symptoms of a low blood glucose level include:

- Shaking or light-headedness

- Nervousness or irritability

- Confusion

- Frequent hunger, even after eating regular meals

- An increase in heart rate

- Sweating or headache onset

- Feeling weak, and/or
- Numbness or tingling on the lips or tongue

If blood glucose level is very low, the ill person will:

- become confused and disoriented
- lose consciousness, and/or
- have a seizure

It is important to respond quickly to a low level of blood glucose. The ill person will likely need assistance in the above situations. It is very important that he/she always wear a MedicAlert identification so that emergency personnel and other people will understand his/her symptoms, and be able to help. People with diabetes (possibly with help from family members) should immediately test their blood glucose level if a low level is suspected. If that isn't possible, it is still better to react immediately to treat the problem. The ill person should do one of the following:

- Eat five glucose tablets
- Drink 3/4 cup of juice OR regular soft-drink
- Eat eight lifesavers or five hard candies, or
- Eat three teaspoons of honey

If after ten to fifteen minutes, there is no improvement:

- Check the blood glucose level again with the meter
- Treat again by eating or drinking something from the list above
- Have a snack that combines carbohydrate and protein (e.g., cheese and crackers, or half of a sandwich)
-

BE PREPARED! It is important to discuss prevention and emergency treatment with a trained health professional. Both the ill person and family members should know how to respond to a situation involving low blood glucose levels. It is a good idea for the ill person to carry glucose tablets or hard candies on him/her at all times.

If the person experiences high blood glucose levels, it is important to call or visit his/her physician. High blood glucose levels can occur when food intake, activity, and medications are not in balance. They may also occur when the person is sick or experiencing more stress than normal. Signs that blood glucose levels are high include an increase in thirst; more frequent urination, and/or an increase in fatigue. The physician may have to adjust medication and/or insulin, recommend a change in diet; or suggest that physical activity be increased.

When the person with diabetes gets sick (e.g., with flu, colds, or any other illness), it is very important that he/she continues to take his/her diabetes medication. Also, he/she should talk to a pharmacist before taking any medication to treat the illness.

When you are sick, it is very important that you:

• Drink plenty of extra sugar-free fluids or water

• Replace solid food with fluids that have glucose if you can't eat as much as normal – try to drink/eat ten grams of carbohydrate every hour

• Call your physician, or go to a hospital if you vomit more than twice in a twelve hour period, and

• Continue to take prescribed insulin – you may need to take more than usual depending on blood glucose levels

Other tips for people with diabetes:

• Don't smoke

• Visit the dentist regularly, and

• Visit the eye specialist at least once every two years

Diabetic Ketoacidosis

A condition known as diabetic ketoacidosis is a potential side effect of atypicial antipsychotic medications. Studies have shown that patients who are male, around the age of forty, non-Caucasian and who take atypical antipsychotics (particularly clozapine and olanzapine) may be at risk. It is essential, therefore, that people with schizophrenia who are treated with clozapine or olanzapine have their blood glucose levels monitored regularly.

Ketoacidosis is a severe and life-threatening complication of diabetes that is the result of high blood sugar levels and ketones. It often arises when diabetes is not properly controlled, or when other illnesses occur. Ketoacidosis usually develops slowly, but if vomiting occurs it can develop in a few hours, possibly causing coma or even death. People with diabetes and their family members should watch for these symptoms:

Symptoms of Diabetic Ketoacidosis Early signs:

- Thirst or a very dry mouth
- Frequent urination
- High blood sugar levels, and/or
- High levels of ketones in the urine

Later signs:

- Constant fatigue
- Dry or flushed skin
- Nausea, vomiting, abdominal pain, or general muscle pains
- Difficulty breathing (short, deep breaths)
- Fruity odour on the breath, and/or
- Confusion or difficulty focusing

If these symptoms appear, the ill person should be seen immediately by a physician for treatment.

It is important to remember that diabetes is a serious illness. It can, however, be controlled through proper management and treatment. Family members may need to pay extra attention to the physical well being of a person with schizophrenia who has diabetes. Diligence is required to ensure the ill person eats regularly and properly, and maintains a healthy lifestyle.

SMOKING AND SCHIZOPHRENIA

Tobacco smoking is a common habit for people with schizophrenia.
Fifty to ninety percent of people with the disorder are smokers (as compared to twenty-five to thirty-five percent of the general population in the United States). More than sixty percent of excess deaths among people with schizophrenia are related to smoking.

One of the reasons smoking may be so popular with people who have schizophrenia is that smoking may lessen the negative symptoms of the illness, and improve the processing of auditory stimuli. This is due to the effect nicotine has on dopamine activity in the brain. Another reason that smoking may be so popular among people with schizophrenia is that it makes them feel more comfortable in social settings.

Smoking increases the metabolism of antipsychotic drugs, and ill individuals who smoke may need higher doses of medicine to control their illness. Higher doses of antipsychotics, however, lead to an increased susceptibility of weight gain, dyslipidemia, hypertension, and diabetes.

Studies show that people who are treated with old or typical antipsychotic drugs tend to smoke more than those who undergo newer or atypcial antipsychotic therapy.

Smoking has very serious, and even deadly, consequences.

Smoking is strongly linked to cardiovascular disease, lung diseases, cancers, and many other serious ailments. People with schizophrenia who smoke are advised to quit this deadly habit. Any gratification that the smoker enjoys is highly outweighed by the negative risks involved. Members of the treatment team may be able to offer suggestions on methods for quitting smoking. Also, smoking cessation programs for hospital outpatients of schizophrenia may be available in your community.

KEY MESSAGES

•   Medical comorbidity of schizophrenia is a serious matter due to its prevalence and its nature

•   It is important that ill individuals and their family members be educated about related illnesses. Be aware of the signs and symptoms that indicate problems such as obesity, heart disease, and diabetes

•   Ensure that either the psychiatrist or a family physician is looking out for medical comorbidity in the person with schizophrenia

•   It is important that people with schizophrenia live a healthy lifestyle to prevent comorbid disease

•   It is necessary that ill people have regular medical check-ups, and be tested for risk factors of comorbid conditions

•   People who do have a comorbid condition (e.g., obesity, cardiovascular disease, diabetes) need to be diligent about their health and lifestyle, and need to be monitored by a physician ●

CHAPTER 10: Living With Schizophrenia

WHAT IT IS LIKE TO HAVE SCHIZOPHRENIA

Testimony of a Person with Schizophrenia

Despite her illness Janice Jordan has successfully accomplished work as an Engineering and Technical Editor for over 20 years and has completed a book of poetry based on her thoughts and experiences.

"The schizophrenic experience can be a terrifying journey through a world of madness no one can understand, particularly the person traveling through it. It is a journey through a world that is deranged, empty, and devoid of anchors to reality. You feel very much alone. You find it easier to withdraw than cope with a reality that is incongruent with your fantasy world. You feel tormented by distorted perceptions. You cannot distinguish what is real from what is unreal. Schizophrenia affects all aspects of your life. Your thoughts race and you feel fragmented and so very alone with your craziness..."

"I have suffered from schizophrenia for over 25 years. In fact, I can't think of a time when I wasn't plagued with hallucinations, delusions, and paranoia. At times, I feel like the operator in my brain just doesn't get the message to the right people. It can be very confusing to have to deal with different people in my head. When I become fragmented in my thinking, I start to have my worst problems. I have been hospitalized because of this illness many times, sometimes for as long as 2 to 4 months.

I guess the moment I started recovering was when I asked for help in coping with the disorder. For so long, I refused to accept that I had a serious mental illness. During my adolescence, I thought I was just strange. I was afraid all the time. I had my own fantasy world and spent many days lost in it.

I had one particular friend. I called him the Controller. He was my secret friend. He took on all of my bad feelings. He was the sum total of my negative feelings and my paranoia. I could see him and hear him, but no one else could.

The problems were compounded when I went off to college. Suddenly, the Controller started demanding all my time and energy. He would punish me if I did something he didn't like. He spent a lot of time yelling at me and making me feel wicked. I didn't know how to stop him from screaming at me and ruling my existence. It got to the point where I couldn't decipher reality from what the Controller was screaming. So I withdrew from society and reality. I couldn't tell anyone what was happening because I was so afraid of being labeled as crazy. I didn't understand what was going on in my head. I really thought that other normal people had Controllers too.

While the Controller was his most evident, I was desperately trying to earn my degree. The Controller was preventing me from coping with everyday events. I tried to hide this illness from everyone, particularly my family. How could I tell my family that I had this person inside my head, telling me what to do, think, and say? It was becoming more and more difficult to attend classes and understand the subject matter. I spent most of my time listening to the Controller and his demands. I really don't know how I made it through college…

Since my degree was in education, I got a job teaching third grade. That lasted about 3 months, and then I ended up in a psychiatric hospital for 4 months. I just wasn't functioning in the outside world. I was very delusional and paranoid, and I spent much of my time engrossed with my fantasy world and the Controller.

My first therapist tried to get me to open up, but… I didn't trust her and couldn't tell her about the Controller. I was still so afraid of being labeled crazy. I really thought that I had done something evil in my life and that was why I had this craziness in my head. I was deathly afraid that I would end up like my three uncles, all of whom had committed suicide. I didn't trust anyone. I thought perhaps I had a special calling in life; something beyond normal. Even though the Controller spent most of the time yelling his demands, I think I felt blessed in some strange way. I felt above normal. I think I had the most difficulty accepting that the Controller was only in my world and not in

everyone else's world. I honestly thought everyone could see and hear him… I thought the world could read my mind and everything I imagined was being broadcast to the entire world. I walked around paralyzed with fear… my psychosis was present at all times. At one

point, I would look at my coworkers and their faces would become distorted. Their teeth looked like fangs ready to devour me. Most of the time I couldn't trust myself to look at anyone for fear of being swallowed.

I had no respite from the illness... I knew something was wrong, and I blamed myself. None of my siblings have this illness, so I believed I was the wicked one.

I felt like I was running around in circles, not going anywhere but down into the abyss of craziness. I couldn't understand why I had been plagued with this illness. Why would God do this to me? Everyone around me was looking to blame someone or something. I blamed myself. I was sure it was my fault because I just knew I was wicked. I could see no other possibilities...

I do know that I could not have made it as far as I have today without the love and support of my family, my therapists, and my friends. It was their faith in my ability to overcome this potentially devastating illness that carried me through this journey. So many wonderful medications are now available to help alleviate the symptoms of mental illness. It is up to us, people with schizophrenia, to be patient and to be trusting. We must believe that tomorrow is another day, perhaps one day closer to fully understanding schizophrenia, to knowing its cause, and to finding a cure..."

—Janice C. Jordan. From <u>Adrift In An Anchorless Reality</u> Schizophrenia Bulletin, Volume 21, No. 3, 1995

EFFECT ON FAMILY MEMBERS

"The typical family of a mentally ill person is often in chaos. Parents look frantically for answers that usually can't be found. Hope turns to despair, and some families are destroyed no matter how hard they try to survive."

– Parent of a child with schizophrenia

When a family learns that their child has schizophrenia, their emotions are similar to those experienced when a major illness, catastrophe, or accident occurs. They feel shocked, sad, angry, and dismayed. Some affected families have described their feelings as follows:

Sorrow – "We feel like we lost a child."

Anxiety – "We're afraid to leave him alone or hurt his feelings."

Fear – "Will we be safe from physical harm? Will the ill person harm himself or herself?"

Shame and guilt – "Are we to blame? What will people think?"

Feelings of isolation – "No one can understand."

Bitterness – "Why did this happen to us?"

Ambivalence toward the afflicted person – "We love him a great deal but when his disability causes him to be cruel, we also wish he'd go away."

Anger and jealousy – "Siblings resent the attention given to the ill family member."

Depression – "We can't talk without crying."

Complete denial of the illness – "This can't happen in our family."

Denial of the severity of the illness – "This is only a phase that will pass."

Blaming each other – "If you had been a better parent…"

Inability to think or talk about anything but the illness – "All our lives were bent around the problem."

Marital discord – "My relationship with my husband became cold. I seemed dead inside."

Divorce – "It tears a family apart."

Preoccupation with moving away – "Maybe if we lived somewhere else, things would be better."

Sleeplessness – "I aged double time in the last seven years."

Weight loss – "We have been through the mill, and it shows in our health."

Withdrawal from social activities – "We don't attend family get-togethers."

Excessive searching of the past for possible explanations – "Was it something we did to him?"

Increased drinking/use of tranquilizers – "Our evening drink turned into three or four."

Concern for the future – "What's going to happen after we're gone? Who will take care of the ill person?"

"People do not cause schizophrenia, they merely blame each other for doing so."

Unfortunately, a common tendency is for family members and the afflicted person to blame one another. Moreover, sisters and brothers often share the same shame and fears that their parents do.

In the following story, a parent describes blame and shame from personal experience:

"I have two sons. My older son is 22 and is in an advanced stage of muscular dystrophy. My younger son is 21 and has been diagnosed as chronically mentally ill. The son that is disabled physically has many special needs. He gets emotional support everywhere he turns. His handicap is visible and obvious and the community, family and friends open their hearts to him, and go out of their way to make his life better.

My other son, on the other hand, is misunderstood and shunned by all. He is also terribly disabled but his disability is not visible. His grandparents, aunts, uncles and cousins all think that he's lazy, stupid, weird, and naughty. They suggest that somehow, we have made some terrible mistake in his upbringing. When they call on the phone they ask how his brother is and talk to his brother, but they never inquire as to him. He upsets them. They also wish that he'd go away."

With time, a good understanding of the illness, and support from others who are experiencing the same challenges, family members can learn to share their feelings and stop destructive blame and shame. In the process, many families discover great strength and deep reserves of love for one another.

NEVER BECOME a moth around the flame of self- blame… It can destroy your chance of coping, FOREVER. It can destroy YOU…"

– Dr. Ken Alexander, 14 Principles for the Relatives

IMPACT ON SIBLINGS

All family members are affected when a loved one develops schizophrenia. Once a diagnosis has been made, it is best that parents explain the disorder and its implications on the family's lifestyle. Siblings will need the direction from their parents to help them understand the strange behaviour of their brother or sister. They have likely suspected that something out of the ordinary is happening, and are probably very confused, frustrated, or even frightened. Like the parents, they too are suffering from a sense of loss of someone they love.

Feelings

Parents can expect that their well children are experiencing the following feelings:

Guilt – knowing their own lives are better than their ill siblings;

Fear and anxiety – that they themselves will develop the illness (or that perhaps their offspring will have schizophrenia);

Sadness and grief – for the loss of the person their brother/sister use to be;

Embarrassment – in front of their friends or in public, as a result of their ill sibling's strange behaviour;

Anger and resentment – at the disruption of family life, and the resulting decrease in attention they get from their parents;

Empathy and love – for their ill brother or sister.

Relationships within the Family

The dynamics of the family relationship will undergo some change – it can't be avoided. The best way to deal with this change is to keep the channels of communication open for the benefit of everyone concerned. For example, your well children are likely to notice the anxiety you are feeling as you struggle with your ill child. This may in turn impact their sense of security. They know their ill sibling needs more attention than they do, but emotionally accepting this fact is difficult. They need reassurance that you are okay, and are there for them.

The relationship between siblings who are well may change for the worse or the better following a diagnosis of schizophrenia. The illness may hurt a previously close relationship, particularly where paranoia is present. Conversely, it may bring two siblings who had little interest in one another closer together because the well sibling feels a sense of compassion and commitment toward his/her ill brother or sister.

When a family member develops mental illness, a sibling may react by withdrawing from family interaction. He/she may want to spend more time with friends or doing extra-curricular activities. It is equally possible that the sibling may become more parent-like, deeply involving him/herself with the ill person and his/her illness, and taking on a protective role. It is important that well siblings be encouraged to find a healthy balance between their own lives and their family life.

Coping Strategies for Siblings

The better educated well siblings are about their brother/sister's illness, the better able they are to cope with schizophrenia. If siblings understand the ill loved one's behaviour as a symptom of a brain disorder rather than as intentionally destructive or disruptive, their negative reactions will be tempered.

Parents are encouraged to be forthright and open about schizophrenia. As well, if the person is comfortable talking about his/her illness, well siblings should discuss it with him/her. Openness is more apt to foster a caring environment. Parents are encouraged to listen to their children's concerns about the ill sibling. If they feel understood by you, they can better cope with the situation. Well siblings should also be able to confide in their friends. This will reduce the likelihood of feeling isolated, and thus burdened by the disorder. They may also benefit from seeing a counsellor, or visiting a support group so they can share their experiences, and know they are not alone. It is important that they feel others care about what they, too, are going through.

Well siblings should be encouraged to maintain a relationship with their ill brother or sister. Common interests may still exist, or a sibling can at least be a compassionate ear for their ill sister or brother. It is important that well siblings understand that their brother/sister is still capable of getting enjoyment from life and people, even if they can't express it.

Everyone feels more in control of a situation when they understand it. Ensure that siblings are well informed about their brother/sister's illness, its symptoms, and treatment on an ongoing basis. This will help them to know what to expect from the ill person, and to understand the person's limitations and capabilities.

Coping Strategies for Parents

Well children need the attention and support of their parents on a regular basis. Parents need to recognize that balancing the needs of all their children is extremely challenging. It may help if each spouse takes turns spending time with the well children for a period, and the ill

child other times. If at all possible, solicit the help of other relatives or friends. Allow your well children to decide how involved they want to be with their ill sibling. Forcing the matter will only create a friction that may negatively affect your ill child. It is also a good idea to consider the future care of your ill child. When you are no longer able to take all the responsibility, who will look after his/her interests? Discuss this situation openly with your family. Well siblings should have the opportunity to consider and make informed decisions about how much or little responsibility they are willing to take on, without having to feel guilty about their choices.

LIVING ARRANGEMENTS

There are a number of options for the ill person's living arrangements. They include living: at home with parents, in a group home, in a boarding house, in an apartment, in a room, or in shared accommodations. The level of functionality of the ill person will be a key determinant when examining housing options. It is, therefore, important to understand the level of support or supervision that each option offers. Group homes may vary considerably in the degree of support they offer.

Supervision may range from 24 hours a day to one person dropping in periodically. There may or may not be in-house counselling or life skills training. Rules and policy may vary considerably. It is obviously necessary to know precisely what is offered before you and your relative can make a decision whether a particular group home is appropriate. Boarding houses and shared accommodation may offer little supervision, and housing in the form of an apartment requires an ability to function well in an independent situation. Initially, a considerable degree of family support is advisable.

Because there are usually waiting lists for supportive housing such as group homes, you should place your relative's name on a list as soon as possible, once a mutually satisfactory decision has been reached.

A decision about housing can often be emotional. Contributing families suggest the following guidelines to help you with your decision.

In general, at-home arrangements seem to work best under the following circumstances:

• the ill person functions at a fairly high level, has friendships, and is involved in activities outside the house

• if there are young children, their lives are not negatively affected

• interaction among family members is relaxed, and

• the ill person intends to take advantage of available support services

In general, at-home arrangements are NOT appropriate in the following circumstances:

• the main support person is single, ill, or elderly

• the person with schizophrenia is so seriously ill that there is little or no chance to lead a normal family life

• children become frightened and resentful, and feel like they are living in a hospital

• marital relationships deteriorate

• most family concerns revolve around the person with schizophrenia

• no support services are used, or services are not available, and

• the individual is habitually aggressive, and the threat of violence disturbs the household.

If the ill individual prefers to live at home, the family as a group should have interviews with the therapist to clarify treatment issues. You should keep a record of how the situation works and how all family members are affected. This will help you to evaluate how well things are, or are not, working. The record may also be useful, if needed, to demonstrate to the ill person that a different housing environment is required.

Families often feel very guilty if they must make the decision not to have the ill person live at home; this appears to be especially true for women. If your experience is similar, consider the following comments of a mother who had to make this decision: "A break should be made at some point, and often it is easier for the ill person to adjust to the transition to a group home, boarding home, or whatever, while you are still available to give support and encouragement, as well as your assistance to participate in activities offered in the community.
Otherwise, they will eventually have to make this adjustment without your help."
Consult with a social worker, community resource person, or other appropriate experts regarding the move toward independent living.

INDEPENDENT LIVING

If ill individuals achieve a good level of functional recovery, one of their goals might be to eventually have an independent living
arrangement (once they have attained an appropriate age). You should gradually begin to plant this concept in an ill person's mind. Subtle hints can be dropped such as: "If you decide to live on your own..."; "When you decide to live on your own..."; " When you start to live on your own, you'll need to know how to do your own laundry.";
" When you live on your own, you'll be glad you learned how to use the laundromat." Time should be allotted between progressive statements to allow for digestion and acceptance of the idea. Leaving the family home is difficult, but a necessary part of life for all of us.

Families suggest that at some point you and the ill individual make a commitment about when the move will occur. Work together (with the social worker, if there is one) to set a date that allows plenty of time to seek and approve accommodation. For example, you may come to an agreement that in six months, on May 1, John will be ready to live on his own, in whatever form of housing he and you have decided will be best.

Once the move has been completed, ill persons may feel some resentment about it. It is very important to help them so that they do not feel abandoned by you. You may have to make an extra effort during the first few weeks to reinforce the idea of the move as a positive step.

•   Be a friend. Call and visit the ill person often, and make dates to go places and do things

•   Encourage self-esteem by offering praise and support

•   Respect the ill person's wishes and concerns as much as possible

As well as emotional support, you may have to get involved in such things as housework, shopping, cooking, and management of finances. The amount of daily assistance the ill person needs will, of course, depend on the condition of his/her illness. Families stress the importance of working with the ill individual as you do these tasks.

Allowing for your family's background and traditions, the relationship should become less intense over time. At first the person may wish to come home every weekend. This is fine for the first few weeks or months. Then, however, you should begin to pick the occasional weekend when he/she will not return home. You should have a valid reason, such as "We'll be away that weekend." Gradually decrease visits to one or two weekends a month. You may also find that at first, the ill person will phone home constantly, often three or four times a day. If this persists, the use of an answering machine may be advisable. You can then return phone calls as you deem appropriate. As time passes, the person should become more confident and comfortable with his/her living arrangement, and the number of phone calls and visits should settle into a normal pattern.

DRUGS & ALCOHOL

It is advisable to have a frank discussion with the ill person about the risks associated with drugs and alcohol. The approach you take should be consistent with the degree of the ill person's level of maturity. You may wish to consult his/her therapist about the best way to do this.

People with schizophrenia can be highly vulnerable to the temptations of the street. They need to be fully aware that the use of drugs or alcohol can impair the effectiveness of their antipsychotic medication. Consumption of street drugs or alcohol can create symptoms of psychosis that are difficult to distinguish from those of a psychotic episode caused by schizophrenia. Street drugs taken by injection add the extra danger of possible infection by the virus that causes AIDS (Acquired Immunodeficiency Syndrome) and/or Hepatitis C.

For more information on the effects of alcohol and street drugs on the recovery process, please refer to Chapter 17, Research, Alcohol/Drugs Recovery,

SEXUALITY, FAMILY PLANNING, PREGNANCY & PARENTING

"No one ever asks us about this (sex). There is the assumption that because I have schizophrenia, I shouldn't have a sex life".

– Anonymous woman with schizophrenia

Historically, the sexual health of individuals with schizophrenia has received little attention from clinicians and researchers. Still, it is well accepted that the illness and the antipsychotics used to treat it can cause sexual problems in both sexes. These include diminished desire, problems with obtaining and/or maintaining an erection, vaginal
dryness, abnormal ejaculation, and orgasmic dysfunction.[20]

Having schizophrenia does not eliminate sexual feelings (although they may be altered during the illness). Sexual side effects can be of great

concern to the person experiencing them, and can also be a key reason for not complying with drug therapy. It is usually during the recovery phase that sex becomes an issue. For example, a sexual relationship that existed prior to the illness will often be put on hold during the acute phase. As symptoms of the illness abate, and the ill person begins to recover, interest in a romantic relationship may be revived. Interest in sexual activity may signal resumption of normal development, as the ill person regains his/her identity and is prepared to seek close relationships again. Successful resumption of sexual activity can help to facilitate the establishment of intimate adult relationships.

It is important to developmental recovery that people with schizophrenia be educated about sexual side effects that can occur, and that they report them to their physician(s). Doctors should actively question patients about sexual side effects of medication. The impact of the side effect on ill persons should be explored. Treatment options should be openly discussed with ill individuals, so that they understand the costs and benefits of potential solutions to the problem. It is possible, for example, that by reducing the dose of antipsychotic medication, the side effect may decrease. It may also be feasible to try different medications. This may be helpful since not all medications cause the same severity of sexual side effects, and ill individuals may be sensitive to side effects from some drugs more than others. It is most important that people with schizophrenia realize that there are ways of treating sexual side effects without ceasing drug treatment for their disorder.

Antipsychotic medications, along with the illness itself, can both affect sexual thoughts and activity. This intimate area of human functioning may be difficult for individuals to discuss, but being open about such concerns can not only greatly reduce them, but lead to solutions that improve quality of life.

SEXUALITY AND MULTICULTURAL ISSUES

Sexuality is viewed differently by different cultures. Pre-marital sex, in particular, is frowned upon by some ethnic groups. Arranged marriages are still prevalent among many cultures. Thus the ill person's background must be carefully considered when it comes to sex. Clinicians and other caregivers should be aware of their patients' values on this issue, and ensure that while hospitalized, he/she is not subjected to sexual advances by other patients. This protection is necessary to uphold the ill person's family traditions, and his/her self-respect.

WOMEN & SEXUALITY

Gender differences affect the impact schizophrenia has on women and men. Women with schizophrenia often have greater social functioning recovery. They spend less time in hospitals[21], and have better chances of social integration in society. For example, they date, have active sex lives, get married, and raise children in greater numbers than their male counterparts. (This is largely attributable to the fact that women tend not to get the illness at very young ages as men do, and their social skills are often well developed by the time they experience schizophrenia.) While women with schizophrenia may have the advantage of better social functioning, the resulting risks can pose serious problems. They become vulnerable to coerced sex, sexually transmitted diseases, and unwanted pregnancies. It is, therefore, important to ensure ill individuals are educated on family planning matters.

FAMILY PLANNING

Statistics reveal that, due to a basic lack of knowledge about contraception, many women who suffer from serious mental illness and are sexually active, do not practice birth control, even though they do not want to become pregnant.[22] Mental health professionals should provide their patients with family planning counselling, but it is not yet common practice. It is a good idea to seek out this service, where available, in order that the person receives psychosocial skills training to reduce the possibility of pressured sex, and to understand the various methods of contraception.

Schizophrenia poses a challenge for women who wish to use contraceptives. Women who use intrauterine devices (IUD's) and other contraceptive implants, face two significant risks: 1) that the devices may become a focus of delusions of control;[23] 2) if the disease interferes with pain perception, the ill person may not recognize early signs of pelvic inflammatory disease caused by the device[24].

Oral contraceptives are difficult for many women to remember. They also affect mood in some people with schizophrenia. Condoms are only effective if the ill person understands proper usage, but will not provide protection in the many instances of unplanned or pressured sex. Often the optimal choice of contraceptive is long acting hormone injections. They usually last three months and do not have any clinically significant interactions with anti-psychotic medication.

PREGNANCY

For women with schizophrenia, pregnancy is a complicated situation. The first problem involves drug therapy. The risks of discontinuing antipsychotic medication must be weighed against its effects on the fetus. An estimated sixty-five percent of patients who discontinue drug therapy while pregnant suffer a relapse during the pregnancy.[25] A state of psychosis will then impair the woman's ability to properly care for herself and her unborn baby. Her stress levels are likely to be high and she may not eat well. As well, the risks of violence, suicide, premature self- delivery attempts, or precipitous delivery are very significant during acute psychotic episodes. There are potential lasting effects on a woman who stops treatment for schizophrenia, since it is consistency of drug therapy that results in significantly better recovery over the ill person's lifetime.

Due to the grave risks of discontinuing antipsychotic treatment, it is important that the ill person and his/her family be well informed about the various psychotropics and their known effects on the fetus. Several studies on the risks to offspring have been performed, and your physicians should have knowledge of available data. In order to make a reasonable risk-benefit analysis that will aid the decision process, ask the doctor(s) about antipsychotic agents and congenital anomalies, fetal development, malformed babies, enduring behavioural changes in offspring, and any other neonatal side effects of antipsychotics, and any other drugs for side effects.

In her article Sexuality, Reproduction, and Family Planning (published in Schizophrenia Bulletin, Vol. 23, No. 4, 1997), Laura J. Miller outlines the steps your physician should be considering when a female with schizophrenia becomes pregnant:

•   Review the available data on prescribing antipsychotic medications during pregnancy

•   Evaluate the risks of both withholding and continuing psychotropic treatment

•   Establish the ill person's capacity to understand this risk-benefit analysis and participate meaningfully in a decision about drug therapy

•   For ill individuals who are unable to give informed consent, pursue the involvement of someone authorized to act on the ill person's behalf, e.g., a guardian or court appointed temporary guardian

•   Once a decision to continue antipsychotic treatment is made, the physician should, wherever possible, prescribe only one neuroleptic (since the effects of drug interactions during pregnancy are unknown)

•   Drugs that will be given priority as a result of study information are trifluoperazine and haloperidol. They appear to have the least risk of neonatal side effects and lasting behavioural implications from receptors

•   Evaluate the use of drugs used to combat neuroleptic side effects, e.g., drugs used to treat EPS pose additional risks during pregnancy.

Akathisia may be safely and effectively treated with beta blocking agents.Neuroleptic malignant syndrome may be treated with supportive measures

• Promote careful attention to nutrition, (e.g., low calcium levels in women with schizophrenia can predispose them to EPS) and prenatal vitamin supplements

• The doctor should make well known to the ill person the additional risks of cigarette smoking while taking neuroleptics during pregnancy, e.g., the increased risk of lower birth weights, and higher morbidity and mortality rates

It is important to realize that challenges of pregnancy to women with schizophrenia do not end with childbirth. The postpartum period presents a high risk for psychosis. Studies show that twenty-four percent

of women become acutely psychotic within six months of childbirth, and forty-four percent whose history included more than three months of hospitalization were subjected to a worsening of symptoms.

The implications of postpartum problems extend to the mother and child relationship. Acute symptoms may include delusions, e.g., that the birth never occurred, or that the baby is dead, or hallucinations, e.g., commanding the mother to harm the baby.[28] Where hospitalization is necessary, new mothers tend to avoid inpatient care because they don't want to be separated from the baby. Another key danger is that the symptoms will be sufficiently severe to cause the mother to neglect caring for herself and her baby, and she may forget to attend pediatric, obstetric, and other medical appointments.

While the new mother with schizophrenia should resume her drug therapy following delivery, she will want to avoid sedating medications, particularly if the baby is breast fed, as they may sedate the baby, or render the mother unable to hear the child crying during the night.

The stress involved in being a new mother, combined with sleep deprivation may be overwhelming for a person with schizophrenia. The addition of psychotic symptoms exacerbates an already difficult situation. Special care must be taken during the postpartum period to ensure the mother is coping with her baby's care, along with her own. Ongoing medical care can help to address problems as they arise, especially if it provides the mother with continued access to her child.

PARENTING

The prospect of parenting poses complex challenges to a person with schizophrenia. Besides the financial burden involved in raising a child, the parent with schizophrenia may be disadvantaged by the disorder in some of the following ways:

•   Reduced ability to understand facial expressions and nonverbal cues from children

•   Reduced ability to provide stability, nurturing, and stimulation of the child

•   Impaired behavioural responses that may cause excessive distancing from the baby or excessive involvement with the child

•   Decreased ability to distinguish their own needs from those of their children

•   Compared to the general population, mothers with schizophrenia are less likely to be married or cohabiting at the time of childbirth, or to have someone to help them raise the child.[29] If married, there is a higher chance that the spouse also has a psychiatric disorder. In either case, the result is a lack of needed parental support for the child

•   The majority of mothers with schizophrenia will experience loss of child custody.[30] Often this will occur intermittently with periods of visits and regaining custody. If loss of custody becomes permanent, it can have devastating results for many women[31]

•   There is some evidence that the children themselves will be more difficult to raise as they may not interact well with others and can be more difficult to deal with than children of mothers who are not mentally ill[32]

For the child, there are risks both in remaining with a parent who is acutely psychotic, and in being separated from the parent. It is believed that children are generally better off remaining with the ill
parent except in instances of child abuse or gross neglect. If a mother with schizophrenia has the support of her family, spouse, and/or extended family connections along with a good comprehensive treatment plan, the prospects of good parenting are much improved.

INTIMATE RELATIONSHIPS

People with schizophrenia may have difficulty maintaining intimate relationships. Marital relationships that involve a spouse with schizophrenia seem to be significantly susceptible to breakdown because couples lack the specialized coping skills required to deal with the disorder. People with schizophrenia also find it difficult to start intimate relationships because they are isolated from the social streams that young people use to meet potential mates. In particular, men who experience schizophrenia often feel they have a disadvantage when it comes to attracting female partners.

Family members can help the ill person by encouraging him/her to get involved in peer support groups, church social groups, or other community groups where he/she can interact with similar others. The treatment team can also help the ill person to develop the social skills he/she requires to socialize with others (see Chapter 7, Treatment, section on Social Skills Training, p. 109 for more information). With support from family and friends, the ill person can pursue intimate relationships.

ELDERLY PEOPLE WITH SCHIZOPHRENIA

Elderly people with schizophrenia often take several medications for various physical conditions, along with anti-psychotic drugs. Extra attention to medication is required, therefore, to ensure that there will be no complications with drug interactions. As well, the type of medication being used should be reviewed for its side effects on geriatric patients. It is possible that dosage levels may be reduced as the ill person gets older and exhibits continued stabilization.

Ensure the elderly person receives proper medical reassessments for schizophrenia, concurrent physical illnesses, sensory deficits, and

medication side effects. ●

CHAPTER 11: Coping With Schizophrenia

ROLE OF THE FAMILY

•	Provide plenty of support and loving care for ill individuals. Help them to accept the diagnosis. Show by your attitudes and behavior that there is hope, the disorder can be managed, and life can be satisfying and productive

•	Help the person with the illness to maintain a record of information on what symptoms have appeared; what medications were taken and in what dosages, and the effects of various types of treatment

•	Ensure that the person continues to receive treatment after hospitalization. This includes taking medication; keeping doctors' appointments; going for follow-up treatment, and participating in social, recreational and vocational programs

•	Provide a structured and predictable environment. The recovering individual will have problems with sensory overload. In order to reduce stress, plan activities for each day and keep big events to a minimum. Keep routines simple and allow the ill person time alone each day

•	Be consistent. Caregivers should agree on a plan of action and follow it. If you are predictable in the way you handle recurring concerns, you will help to reduce confusion and stress for the ill person

•	Maintain peace and calm at home. You will want to keep voices down and speak at a slower pace. Shorter sentences will also help to reduce stress. Avoid arguing about delusions (false beliefs)

•	Be positive and supportive. Being positive will probably be more helpful and effective in the long run than criticism. Like anyone else, people with schizophrenia need to know when they are doing well. Their self-esteem is fragile and needs to be boosted regularly. Encourage all positive efforts. Express appreciation for a job even half-done because schizophrenia creates a lack of confidence, initiative, patience, and memory

•	Assist the ill person to set realistic goals. Encourage him/her to gradually regain former skills and interests. Try new things as well, but work up to them gradually. If goals are unattainable or if you nag, stress can worsen the symptoms

• Gradually increase independence when the ill person shows the ability to handle greater responsibility and is able to complete various types of chores. Set limits on how much abnormal behaviour is acceptable and firmly and consistently apply the consequences. As well, some re-learning may have to occur about the handling of money, cooking and housecleaning. If outside employment is too difficult, help the person learn how to use time constructively

• Together learn how to cope with stress. Anticipate ups and downs and prepare accordingly. A person with schizophrenia needs to learn to deal with stress in a socially acceptable manner. Your positive role modeling will be most helpful

• Encourage the ill individual to get out into the community. Allow him/her to participate in the selection of an appropriate activity when trying something new. If requested, go along the first time for moral support

• Be good to yourself. Your good health is very important, even crucial, to the best functioning of your entire family. Let go of guilt and shame. Take comfort and gain strength from the positive things your family has experienced together

• Establish realistic expectations and goals for yourself within your own life. Make sure you are allotting yourself time for extra- curricular activities, hobbies, physical exercise/sports, etc. You need time for yourself in order to rejuvenate and maintain the stamina necessary to help others

• Value your own privacy. Keep up friendships and outside interests and lead as orderly a life as possible

• Do not neglect other children. Brothers and sisters often secretly share the guilt and fear of their parents. They may worry that they too may become ill. When their concerns are neglected because of the ill child, they can become jealous or resentful. These children need your love and attention, too

• Learn from and enjoy the support of others who have similar problems. Check to see what resources are available in your community. You can share and learn from the experiences of others, you can benefit from educational programs and discussions, and you can work cooperatively with others to improve and increase services

• Call the Mental Health Clinic in your region and ask if there is a family or parent education program that you can join

• Join the Schizophrenia Society of Canada and one of its local chapters, or similar family support organization in your region. These community resources offer support, education, help and hope to families who may be experiencing a crisis

ENCOURAGING MEDICATION

This is one of the most frustrating problems. It may be hard to understand why someone with schizophrenia would refuse to take medication when its necessity is so obvious to everyone else.

Families have found that there are five main reasons why someone might refuse medication:

1. The ill person may lack insight about the illness. Not believing that he/she is ill, he/she sees no reason to take medication. Or, some think that it is the medication that causes the illness. If the illness involves paranoia, the ill individual may view the medication as part of a plot to prevent him/her from functioning

2. The ill person may be suffering from unpleasant side effects as a result of the medication and believe that it causes more problems than it solves

3. The person may be on a complicated medication scheme that involves taking several pills a day. He/she may find the regimen too confusing, and may resent the constant reminders of illness

4. The ill person may feel so well that he/she either forgets to take the medication, or think that it is not necessary any more

5. The ill individual may welcome the return of particular symptoms such as voices that say nice things and make him/her feel special

People with schizophrenia need to take prescribed medication, and the following is a list of ideas and guidelines to help you encourage drug therapy:

• The initial medication dose must be continuously monitored. Therefore, you should always listen to the ill person's complaints about side effects. Do your best to empathize with any distress about medications

• Positive symptoms will not reappear immediately upon discontinuation of medication. Antipsychotic drugs stay in the system for six weeks to three months. This grace period gives you some time to deal with the problem. After three months, however, getting back to a maintenance level may mean starting over at a higher than maintenance dosage

•   Explain to the person that he/she may end up back in the hospital if medication is not taken (this should not be a threat). Some people will not accept warnings, and still others may not mind returning to the hospital

•   If other people in your family are on medication, turn pill taking into a ritual. Everyone could take their medication at the same time (even if it is a vitamin pill). It is easier to take one pill a day than six. Talk to the doctor about the form in which the ill person is receiving medication

•   For people who keep forgetting to take oral medication, the use of a weekly pill box can be an effective tool

•   Never sneak pills into food. If paranoia exists, this will increase it. Trust will never be established

•   More people go off oral medication than injectable medication. With injections, you are sure the person is getting his/her medicine. He/she can't spit it out, hide it under the tongue, etc. Discuss the pros and cons of switching medications with the doctor. (Health care professionals note that there is a down side to injections: possible feelings of humiliation, loss of control, and the potential for build-up of medication over time.)

•   Injectable medication is given once a week or once every few weeks, depending on the type of antipsychotic. Consider arranging a treat built around going for the medication – seeing a movie, going for lunch, etc. Let the ill person know that you are proud of the way in which he/she is handling the need for medication

Do your best to be calm and reasonable about getting the ill person to take medication. If you push too hard, you may make it more difficult for him/her to move to greater independence. A period of learning through experience may be necessary.

LEGAL ISSUES

MENTAL HEALTH LEGISLATION

All provinces and territories in Canada have mental health legislation, usually referred to as Mental Health Acts. There are two key objectives to these laws:

1   to protect the legal rights of a person with a severe mental illness, and

2   to help provide treatment to a person with a severe mental illness who refuses needed treatment, and who is likely to suffer harm or cause harm to others.

Since mental health legislation differs from province to province, the information provided here is general. The degree and type of harm criterion that a person must meet before becoming an involuntary patient is specific to each province. A few provinces restrict the definition of harm to mean physical bodily harm. Most provinces, however, include serious non-physical harms in their criterion for involuntary patients. Some provinces have a broader definition of harm that includes significant mental or physical deterioration of the ill person. It is a good idea to consult your provincial Schizophrenia
Society and a knowledgeable mental health or legal professional about the law in your province.

Involuntary Admission Procedures

(i)   Physician Certificates

If the ill person will not go to the hospital voluntarily, but a medical examination performed by a physician determines he/she meets the criterion for involuntary admission, then this is the preferable method to enforce hospitalization. In most provinces one physician can, upon examination, issue a certificate that authorizes the transportation and admission to hospital for a short period of time (e.g., 1-3 days). A few Canadian provinces require two physician's certification to enforce hospital admission. A second certificate is required to hospitalize the person for an additional period of time (e.g., two weeks to one month), and this may be granted upon examination in the hospital.

(ii)   Judge's Order

If the ill person refuses to allow a physician to examine him/her, then any person can go to a judge and apply for the compulsory psychiatric examination of another person. Mental health laws require that if such an order is requested, it must be accompanied by evidence that shows the ill person is suffering from a mental disorder, is refusing to see a physician, and meets criteria for harm, danger, or safety concerns as specified by the provincial legislation. If the judge is satisfied that the criterion for involuntary examination are met, the court can order the transportation and physical examination of the ill person. The results of the medical examination may then lead to involuntary hospitalization.

(iii)   Police Apprehension

There are times, such as emergency situations, when it is not practical to use a physician or judge to enforce hospitalization of the ill person. The police may be your only resort in a time of crisis. Mental health legislation does give the police the authority to apprehend a person if the person meets the criterion for police enforcement (e.g., appear to be ill and in danger). The police may take the ill person to have a medical examination, which in turn may lead to involuntary hospitalization.

Legal Rights and Protections While in Hospital

When a person is involuntarily detained in accordance with provincial mental health laws, the Charter of Rights and Freedoms (of Canada) requires that the ill person be informed of certain rights. For example, the right to be told of the reason for his/her detention, and the right to consult a lawyer. In addition, Mental Health Acts provide further rights such as the right to a review board to determine if the person can be released; the right to have regular examinations (renewal certificates), and in some cases, the right to have second medical opinions on the appropriateness of the medical treatment.

Family Involvement

In this book, we emphasize the importance of family involvement to help the ill person during acute episodes, and throughout the course of the illness. We have also talked about the importance of working closely with the treatment team. Specific opportunities for family involvement are provided by most provincial mental health legislation. They include:

•   The family's right to provide information to a judge to facilitate admission to hospital

•   The family or next of kin are supposed to be notified that the ill person has been involuntarily admitted to hospital, and given information about family and patient rights

• In some provinces, treatment can be authorized by the hospital, but in the majority of provinces it is a family member or next of kin who must authorize treatment. Some provinces (e.g., Alberta) dictate that the family member who authorizes the treatment must act in the person's best interests. In Ontario, this is also the practice with the exception that if there are prescribed treatment wishes as set out by the ill person while he/she was still competent, those wishes must be granted. Families should be aware that if they refuse to authorize treatment as recommended by the hospital, then the ill person may continue to suffer and be detained in hospital unnecessarily

• Most provincial mental health legislation provides that families must be informed when an involuntary patient applies to a medical review board (tribunal, or panel) to be released from hospital, or to

change/review some other treatment decision. Families are usually given the opportunity to give evidence to the board that will be considered in the decision process

• Provinces that have conditional leave or community treatment order provisions allow the families to be involved in the development of the plan. In Ontario, a next of kin must consent to the order if the ill person is not capable

Assisted Community Treatment

Despite the efforts of family and caregivers, some people with schizophrenia discontinue their treatment once they are discharged from hospital. There are various reasons for ill persons to stop medication, but once they have, they are often subjected to relapses and readmission to hospital. This disrupts their lives considerably, and if there are numerous re-admissions, other alternatives may be appropriate. Assisted community treatment measures, including conditional leave from hospital or community treatment orders are available in most provinces to address this problem. Evidence has shown that they are effective in reducing rates of hospitalization.

CONFIDENTIALITY

Sooner or later families run up against the legal and ethical issue of confidentiality. It is a basic principle in the practice of medicine.

Information about a patient cannot usually be released, except to members of the treatment team, unless that patient has given written consent. The exceptions are when a person is under age or is deemed to be mentally incompetent. Under the law of some jurisdictions, a priority list of those who may act on behalf of a mentally incompetent person has been established. It often comes as a surprise to family members that they are not first on such lists. In the case of a spouse in Ontario, if the person who is ill has appointed someone else while still mentally competent, that person ranks before the spouse.

It is natural for caregivers to want to know as much as they can about the ill person's health in order to help as much as possible. Health care professionals recognize this, but their hands may be tied because no patient's consent has been given. Ideally, written authorization for the doctor to talk to the family should be obtained when the patient is well. However, if the ill person is unwilling to give consent, try asking the physician whether there is anything that you can do to help obtain it. Note that a physician can speak if there is a risk of physical violence.

Legal requirements on the release of medical information vary between provinces and territories. You can ask a health care professional what is needed in your particular province or territory. It may be worth seeing if it is possible to attend some of the health care team meetings or consultations with the ill person. The ill person may be more willing to accept this than to sign a consent form for the release of information.

Physicians and other health care professionals will normally look to family members to supply information about the ill person. At the doctor's discretion, this information may be passed on to the ill individual. You may wish to consider, therefore, the effects of telling the ill person directly about any information that you share with a member of the treatment team. Care providers often find that this enhances their caregiving relationship with the ill person.

SSC is currently lobbying the provincial and federal governments to enact legislation entitling family caregivers the right to information on their ill loved ones. The model being advocated is the approach taken by British Columbia. Legislation is needed across the country, providing uniformity for Canadians dealing with confidentiality and mental illness.

ADVICE FROM A CROWN ATTORNEY (PROSECUTOR)

Unfortunately, some people with schizophrenia get in trouble with the law. Offenses may range from minor altercations like shoplifting, mischief, assault, or ordering a meal at a restaurant and refusing to pay for it, to much more serious charges such as aggravated assault, arson, or even murder. These problems arise most commonly when the ill persons are not being medically treated for their disorder. The tragedy that this presents is far too common: a mentally ill person is placed in the criminal justice system instead of being treated in a hospital.

When persons with schizophrenia have to face criminal charges, their illness may mean they are unfit to stand trial, or are not criminally responsible. These are legal concepts that relate to the state of mind of an accused person. Fitness to stand trial is based on the accused's mental capacity to understand the trial process, for example, the ability to instruct a lawyer, understand the role of the Crown Attorney (or Prosecutor), and understand the applicable penalties. Criminal responsibility applies to the accused's state of mind at the time of the offense. The state of mind is tested by his/her awareness of the consequences of his/her actions, and whether or not he/she appreciates the act is morally wrong. For example, could the accused's illness be affecting him/her in such a manner that he/she believes he/she is tickling someone, when in fact he/she is stabbing a person. Or, could it be that voices convince the ill individual to believe that by killing a person, he/she is saving the world from a terrible evil.

If the charge is serious, and the ill person goes through the court process, and is found either unfit to stand trial or not criminally responsible, his/her fate will be determined by a provincial Review Board. The Board includes professionals in the legal field and psychiatric field. If the accused is found unfit to stand trial, this is a temporary status, meaning that he/she must return to court when he/she becomes fit. In the case of either finding, the Board imposes conditions on the accused such as where and under what circumstances he/she may reside; whether or not he/she must be hospitalized, for what duration, and under what conditions the accused may be released from the hospital. If the Board permits the accused to reside in the community, and the accused does not follow the conditions of the court, he/she may be detained. The Board normally reviews the status of the accused once a year at a formal hearing, and family members/ caregivers may attend these hearings and give evidence. If the accused was found not criminally responsible, and the Board concludes that he/she is not a significant threat to the safety of the public, the Board may grant him/her an absolute discharge, thereby ending its jurisdiction over the ill person.

Just because a person has schizophrenia does not mean he/she will automatically be declared unfit to stand trial, or not criminally responsible. It is not the diagnosis that determines his/her status, but to what extent the disorder was affecting him/her at the time of the offense (in the case of criminal responsibility), or at the time of trial (in the issue of fitness to stand trial). Presumably if he/she is not taking his/her medication, he/she is likely being very strongly affected by his/her illness.

If the offense is minor, and the accused is not a risk to public safety, it is feasible — and most preferable — to keep the ill person out of the criminal justice system. This goal may be achieved through a process known as diversion. Diverting the case means to have the criminal charge stayed or withdrawn by the Prosecutor, so that the ill person will not be tried. The decision to divert the case rests with the Crown Attorney's office (or Crown Prosecutor's office), and depends upon a number of factors including the availability of community programs, the extent of family support, the nature of the offense, the effects of the illness, and the disposition of the offender.

Families are advised to explore community programs that support the ill person's case for diversion. For example, there are sponsored court outreach workers in some municipalities who help the accused find an arrangement that will comply with the conditions for diverting his/her criminal charges.

The impact of hospital cutbacks and cuts in social programs in Canada has had a truly tragic impact on the welfare of mentally ill people. The number of patients who become homeless or end up in jail has been steadily increasing over the past few years. If you find yourself faced with legal issues involving an ill person in your care, consider the following suggestions:

•   Seek a lawyer (or legal aid lawyer) who is familiar with the law and the mentally ill. Your local legal aid office, the Canadian Mental Health Association, a psychiatric hospital's forensic department, or police headquarters may be able to provide a list of lawyers who specialize in this area. Be warned that there are not many attorneys with this experience, so your search may require some patience

• If you're hopeful of having the accused released on bail, you should be sure to have a lawyer represent the accused at a Bail Hearing pending his/her trial, or while diversion options are being explored. Also, be prepared to assure the judge that the ill person will be well supervised if released

• If you are seeking to get the case diverted, speak to a lawyer or legal aid duty counsel, if at all possible. If necessary, speak to the Crown Attorney (Prosecutor) or prosecutor handling the case

• The lawyer representing the accused or the Crown Attorney (Prosecutor) may ask the court to make an Assessment Order. This order is applicable where there are grounds to believe a person may be suffering from a mental disorder, and needs to be assessed in order to determine whether or not he/she is fit to stand trial or he/she was criminally responsible at the time of the offense. The order is set for a specific number of days. How the accused is then dealt with depends on your jurisdiction. Problems such as bed shortages and waiting lists for psychiatrists could mean that the ill person ends up sitting in a detention centre instead of being assessed in a hospital or cared for at home. It is therefore preferable for the accused to be remanded out of custody while complying with the assessment order

• Get in touch with a Schizophrenia Society (local chapter, provincial office, or national office). They may be able to direct you to an information centre, or provide you with literature, or recommend resources

WILLS

If the ill person outlives you, you may want to make plans and preparations to provide for him/her. The first and most important piece of advice is to SEEK ASSISTANCE FROM PROFESSIONALS who understand your situation and who know the rules about disability benefits in your province.

Here are some legal and financial tips from families who are experienced in these matters:

• Appoint a trustee for administration of the mentally ill person's inheritance

• Bequeath only financial assets – no real estate or portable items

- Provisions for access to income from investments for the ill person should have a condition attached such that the trustee can withhold and/or administer sufficient money to ensure medications, housing, food, and other basic necessities are provided to the beneficiary. Even if the person is managing on his/her own, this provision protects him/her in the event of relapse

- Provision should be made that the trustee is to access the capital of the trust only if it is deemed necessary for the welfare of the mentally ill individual

- Provision should be made to allow for control of the trust to be relinquished to the ill person should a cure be found for schizophrenia, and psychiatric experts have determined that the ill person has achieved permanent stabilization, and is competent to manage the assets on his/her own

- When the ill person dies, a provision should be made so that the rest and residue of the trust can be passed on to a specified next of kin. If this person predeceases the individual, provision could be made to pass on the balance of the trust to your choice of charities

FINANCES

MANAGING MONEY

Many people with schizophrenia have trouble in handling money matters. This can present families with some awkward situations, some of which may be beyond an immediate solution.

Patients who are entitled to disability benefits can get help to apply for them while still in hospital. Disability benefits are paid on a monthly basis. Most recipients will need a good deal of help learning how to budget properly to meet basic needs such as rent, food, and transportation. They may find it difficult to make the money last for the whole month. When a substantial sum is available (for example, on receipt of a disability cheque), many tend to blow all or a large part on impulse spending, often foolishly, or to give their money away to friends — even to strangers. Families find that they are then called upon to pay for basic living expenses.

Behaviour of this sort, although not surprising for someone with few chances to enjoy life, is disconcerting for families, and requires that they exercise a good deal of patience. For the individual, managing money well is an important step toward the achievement of greater independence. By linking behaviour that demonstrates responsibility (e.g., successful completion of chores) to autonomy in handling money, you may be able to help the ill person learn to manage his/her finances. Here are some ideas on how to make life a little easier on the family while giving the ill person a sense of independence:

• Consider arranging for the disability cheque to be delivered to a parent or guardian

• Investigate the possibility of pre-paying landlords, utility companies etc. so that the ill person's rent, heat, hydro, and phone bills are covered

• Your local grocer may be asked to create vouchers for the ill person, paid for by the family in advance, and redeemable on a weekly basis by the holder

• Arrange with a local restaurant to pay for meals on the ill person's behalf

• Provisions could be made with a local pharmacy, smoke shop, bookstore, etc. so that a debit/credit system for goods is in place for the ill person (e.g., you pay so many dollars which credits his/her account, and purchases made by the ill person are debits against the account). You should, of course, be sure to make your instructions clear as to overdrawing/zero balance accounts

Complete awareness of the arrangements is necessary for the ill individuals to understand, and learn about managing money. Hopefully, they will eventually learn to deal with their finances on their own.

DISABILITY BENEFITS

The provision for disability benefits or allowances comes from provincial governments. Terminology and criteria for financial assistance may vary from province to province. The general concept, however, is based on the level of disability, the age of the disabled person, and the ability of the person to work.

For further information, please contact your local chapter or provincial office of the Schizophrenia Society, or your provincial government.

People involved with schizophrenia find the family, who is most often the primary source of support for the ill person, is under a great deal of stress every day.

"Personal stress is something that often goes unacknowledged. The sick person becomes a priority, and we forget our own needs. The day-to-day tasks involved in caring for a dependent – sudden crises, worry, financial problems, searching for community services, coping with bureaucracy, becoming an advocate, squeezing out precious moments for our other family members – depletes and robs us of our energy. Eventually we end up with stress exhaustion, and this can lead to depression, anxiety, burnout, and psychosomatic illnesses.

Families and health care professionals caution that the strain of having a relative with schizophrenia can begin in the very early days, when that person first behaves unusually. Normally, when we see someone who is visibly handicapped — for example, using a wheelchair or white cane — we are inclined to offer that person our support. With mental illness, however, often the only way we realize that something is wrong is to actually see the person exhibit abnormal behaviour. It is natural to be disturbed by such behaviour, and to tend to withdraw from it. When unusual behaviour occurs within a family, the reaction is not much different, and may even be hostile. In the early days, family members may be bewildered and resentful, and often blame and criticize the ill individual. Members may blame other members of the family as their fear and frustration grows.

Families caution that one of the most important things to watch for is resentment in siblings. When you are spending all of your time and energy supporting and seeking help for your ill child, it is very easy to neglect other children. You may also have to accept that a sibling may never have any feeling of affection for his/her ill brother or sister. As one woman said,

"My brother was several years older than me. I never had a relationship with him when he wasn't ill. When he first got sick, I was very young, and his behaviour scared me. Then, as I got older, the things he did embarrassed me. It's very hard for my parents to accept, but I don't feel any connection to this ill man."

Many parents cannot understand this lack of empathy, and find that they resent their other children for not feeling the same way they do about the ill individual. Some families believe that one way to prevent resentment is to include siblings in family discussions about the ill relative, and to ask for their support and/or advice regarding care.

Parents often try to protect children by keeping the truth from them, but ignorance can be very frightening. Children should be given as much information as is appropriate for their age. One woman, whose parents always included her in the support of her brother, stated,

"My brother is only one year older than me. I don't remember a time when he wasn't there. I love him dearly, and I am the only person he can really talk to about what is happening to him."

One father remarked that now that his ill daughter is on medication and doing well, his other three daughters are willing to be supportive. In the past, they were afraid of, and embarrassed by, their sister. But now all four girls go out once a week, and have strong family ties.

Because different relationships within a family can be strained during the very early days, families of those with schizophrenia stress again the importance of joining a support group as soon as the diagnosis has been determined. Listening to others who have been through the experience will help you to acknowledge your feelings of anger, confusion, guilt, shame, and so on, and to realize that this is normal.

Normal as these feelings are, however, they are painful and will worsen if the family members are uninformed and unsupported. The sooner a family comes to an understanding of the illness and finds appropriate ways of relating to the ill individual, the greater chance a family has of remaining a healthy, functioning unit.

Another reason for joining a support group early is to find ways of avoiding the burnout that so often comes with the burden of caring for someone with schizophrenia. Feelings of chronic fatigue, a lack of interest in life, a lack of self-esteem, and a loss of empathy for the person with schizophrenia are common to people who have been coping alone for a number of years. These people are the walking wounded, and may suffer from headaches, insomnia, drug and alcohol abuse, depression, and stress-related illnesses.

Families offer the following ideas for avoiding burnout:

• Be aware of your health on a day-to-day basis. Eat nutritiously. Join an exercise club. Go for walks as often as possible. Get enough sleep.

Visit your own doctor for regular check-ups. Let him/her know that you are the caregiver of a person with schizophrenia

• Learn about, and practice, relaxation techniques

• Schedule a break for yourself every day

• Take regular vacations if you can. Try to get a day or a night to yourself every now and then. Perhaps a friend or relative could stay overnight while you go to a hotel

• Avoid self-blame and destructive self-criticism

• Take a school course – give yourself a few hours when you have to concentrate on something else

• If the person with schizophrenia lives away from home, don't visit more than three times a week after the initial transition, and limit phone calls

• Try not to neglect the other relationships in your family

• Share your grief and problems with supportive people

• Aim for teamwork in your family

• Recognize that successful treatment and workable after-care programs require the coordinated and shared efforts of several groups of caregivers

• Realize that life must go on for you and for others in the family. This attitude may benefit the ill individual. He/she may be strengthened by the realization that life goes on

• Keep on top of developments in the ill person's illness that may indicate that a change of lifestyle is necessary. For example, many families find that although their ill relative lived at home successfully for a number of years, at some point a change occurred that lowered the quality of life for everyone. Do not insist on keeping the ill person at home if different housing is now required

• Keep your religious beliefs and family traditions. This may be important to the ill person's sense of continuity and quality of life

• Keep a sense of humour

• Never lose hope

Burnout may also be caused by a lack of acceptance on the family's part. Some people are unable to recognize the illness for what it is. They never let go. They never get on with their own lives. They wear themselves out. Those with experience advise that once you let go, once you say, "This is it", life becomes simpler. One father stated,

"You work through fear, anger, grief, and finally come to acceptance. Acceptance is like adopting someone new – the other person is no longer there."

Acceptance means that you have learned to look at the ill person as he/she is now. Then there is room for hope, and you can begin to work for those things that will really make a difference in his/her life.

ROLE OF EDUCATORS

"Professionals ...must help the ill person set realistic goals. I would entreat them not to be devastated by our illnesses and transmit this hopeless attitude to us. I would urge them never to lose hope, for we will not strive if we believe the effort is futile."

Esso Leete (who has lived with schizophrenia for more than 20 years) now commits herself to educating others about mental illness.

As an educator, you can play an important role in the lives of those living with schizophrenia. Here are some facts you should be aware of:

•   Schizophrenia is a common illness which strikes many young people in their mid to late teens and early twenties

•   Most people with schizophrenia have normal intelligence and many have high I.Q.'s

•   In very rare instances, children between the age of five and adolescence can develop schizophrenia. At this early age, these children are frequently described only as being different from other children; they are unlikely to display psychotic symptoms until adolescence or adulthood

Here are some suggestions on how you can help those living with schizophrenia:

•   Wherever possible, bring the illness into the open. Openly discuss the issues with your students in classes such as Health and the Sciences. Such action can help to dispel some of the myths and reduce the stigma associated with the illness

•   Provide preventive information on precipitating factors such as drug abuse

•   Be alert to the early warning signs of schizophrenia. Young people often have mood swings, become apathetic, and experience a drop in athletic or academic performance, among other things; but if such behavior persists, you may wish to consult with the student's family and assist the young person to receive an assessment

If you have a student in your classroom who has been diagnosed as having schizophrenia, you can:

•   Reduce stress for the young person by slowing your pace when explaining situations that are new to the student

•   Help the young person to set realistic goals for academic achievement and for extracurricular activities

•   Establish ongoing communication with the student's family for feedback on his/her progress. As a result, you may find that in order to optimize the learning situation, you will have to modify learning objectives, content of curricula, teaching methodology, student evaluation format, and other educational concerns

•   Encourage other students to extend their friendship. Some may wish to act as peer supports when illness occurs, perhaps helping the student to catch-up on missed lessons

In the school environment, you can assist families dealing with schizophrenia in the following ways:

•   If you have a peer counselling program in your school, the illness of schizophrenia, as it affects young people and their families, should be one of the special needs areas addressed by the program

•   Ask your education directors to provide training on schizophrenia at professional development sessions

•   Run informational sessions on the illness for parent nights and student assemblies, and set up displays (ask a mental health organization to help you) for special occasions in the school library and counselling office

•   Order print and audiovisual resource materials for your library. Just as you have reference and instructional materials available on other subjects, so you should have materials on schizophrenia

As an educator, you have an excellent opportunity to help alleviate the suffering caused by schizophrenia. We encourage you to participate by fostering understanding and compassion for people with brain disorders.

MISSING PERSONS

Frequently, people with schizophrenia decide that a new location will provide an answer to the problems that the illness has imposed on them – or they may be directed by voices to leave. They simply disappear. If the ill person is a minor, you should contact the Missing Persons Bureau of the local police department. If he/she is legally of age the police may have no authority to return the ill person, or to inform you of his/her actions or whereabouts.

It may happen that the ill person leaves the hospital before treatment has been completed. If the person is an involuntary patient, the hospital is responsible for notifying the police to look for and return the patient to the hospital. In some jurisdictions, if the police have been unable to find a missing involuntary patient within a certain period, the hospital then has the right to discharge the person.

When a person with schizophrenia has disappeared from the hospital, the option of changing the patient's voluntary status to involuntary is open to the attending physician(s). The police can then be asked to look for the patient.

Often, relatives and caregivers may simply have to wait until the ill person surfaces. This may happen when the person has been picked up as a vagrant, has gone to a hostel, or has been taken to a hospital for help. Then, (unless the police have been involved) you may make arrangements for the person to return home or consider other options.

Here are some tips on preparing yourself for a possible disappearance of the ill person:

• If the ill person mentions places he/she is interested in, or would like to visit sometime, jot it down. It could be a useful clue as to where to look should he/she disappear

- If he/she decides to travel, try to think of some effective way of staying in touch. For example, one father arranged with his son that he would keep his son's money for him. Then, whenever the son needed some funds, the father would send him some, but not too much. This was an effective way of maintaining contact

Some ideas to consider if the ill person disappears:

- If you have lost touch with him/her for a period of time, it is wise not to wait too long before you begin checking. Although the police may have no basis for active involvement, it is worth speaking to Missing Persons and telling them your story. They may be able to help by doing some checking, or offering some practical advice

- In 1998, SSC created a working group to develop a Missing Persons Registry. Our hope is that, with the help of volunteers across Canada, and the cooperation of other organizations (e.g., hospitals, governments, coroners' offices), a database may be implemented to track ill individuals as they move within and across provincial boundaries. This project was undertaken in the hopes

of helping people with schizophrenia maintain their medication a nd treatment program while away from home, and to attempt to alleviate some of the fears and worries of family members and caregivers by locating these ill people. If you have some idea where the ill individual may have gone, get in touch with your local Schizophrenia Society chapter or the national office in Markham.

They may be able to help you through a provincial association or chapter in the area where you think the ill person may be.

- If travel to the United States is a possibility, contact the National Alliance for the Mentally Ill (NAMI) directly or through SSC

- Check with local voluntary agencies such as the Salvation Army. Sometimes a missing person will show up in one of their hostels. Also your place of worship may be able to help, particularly if the ill individual took a keen interest in religion

If you decide to use the services of a firm of private investigators, determine if the firm you select is well connected with the police (they may be able to get help from this source that you cannot.) Discuss with the firm a reasonable limit on its expenses, including the

fee, to undertake a realistic search on your behalf. ●

CHAPTER 12: Impaired Cognition In Schizophrenia

Traditionally, functioning of the mind is described under four headings
—   perception, emotion, cognition, and conation. Perception refers to awareness of surroundings, usually through sensory functions such as seeing, hearing, smelling, tasting or touching. Emotions refer to feelings such as happiness, sadness, anger etc. Conation refers to behaviour or actions, e.g., walking, cooking etc. Cognition is derived from the Latin word Cognitio, which means to know. In modern psychology and psychiatry, the phrase "cognitive functions" is used to describe various aspects of thinking such as attention, concentration, comprehension, memory, orientation, abstraction and judgment. Cognitive functions range from simple abilities such as counting change from a dollar, to complex tasks requiring concentration and coordination such as playing chess, driving a car or writing poetry.

IS COGNITION IMPAIRED IN SCHIZOPHRENIA?

The simple answer is yes. However, there are some controversies and caveats about it. The controversies become evident from a historical review of the concept of schizophrenia. At first, pioneering psychiatrists such as Kreapelin and Bleuler believed that schizophrenia, over a period of time, causes a cognitive decline. In the intervening years, others viewed schizophrenia from a narrower perspective, and described it in terms of distorted thoughts (delusions) and perceptual problems (hallucinations) without the involvement of cognitive functions. These views have again changed over the past two decades, and we have now come to believe that cognitive impairment is commonly associated with schizophrenia.

Schizophrenia is now considered to have four sets of symptoms: positive symptoms, negative symptoms, disorganization symptoms, and cognitive deficits. The relationship between cognitive disturbances and other symptoms of schizophrenia is not clearly understood at present. It has been observed that some people experience cognitive problems before they develop positive symptoms, while others acquire cognitive deterioration after the first episode and with subsequent relapses.
The emergence of cognitive deficits, generally speaking, augurs an unfavourable outcome in the long term.

There are two caveats though, to remember. First, there is a great variability in the occurrence of these different sets of symptoms. Some people experience positive symptoms only, while others may have more negative symptoms, and a proportion of affected individuals develop cognitive difficulties. Second, the extent of cognitive involvement may also vary between different individuals. The majority of people diagnosed with schizophrenia experience only subtle difficulties, while a smaller group (about 1 in 5) seem to show more striking cognitive deficits.

HOW DO COGNITIVE PROBLEMS AFFECT DAILY ROUTINE IN SCHIZOPHRENIA?

The person experiencing cognitive difficulties often complains of speeded-up thinking, racing thoughts, feeling mixed up, and having poor concentration or being forgetful (memory problems). When these problems are mild, the person will have difficulties with reading, writing or watching TV. People with a greater degree of cognitive problems will be unable to carry out tasks (e.g., cooking, shopping, etc.), manage their money, and look after themselves. This may result in poor hygiene, malnutrition, and self-neglect. The worst type of cognitive impairment results in potentially dangerous behaviours such as walking into traffic, leaving the stove on, or mixing up medications. Over time, cognitive difficulties lead to consequences such as unemployment, disability, poverty, debts, and excess dependency.

Two of the common and frustrating problems are forgetting to take medications, and neglecting to keep medical appointments.

WHAT CAUSES COGNITIVE DEFICITS IN SCHIZOPHRENIA?

It is now generally believed that schizophrenia is a brain disorder, and the variety of symptoms experienced is the result of an impaired function in different parts of the brain. The part of the brain located in the forehead (the frontal lobes) holds the key to many cognitive functions. Recent research indicates that other structures located deep inside the brain may also be involved. Damaged nerve cells (neurons) located in these parts interfere with the transmission of information from one part of the brain to the other (neuronal circuits), produce a chemical imbalance, and lead to cognitive decline. Some of the speculated mechanisms include an inability to distinguish between useful and useless information (filtering), resulting in an information overload; failure to have a working memory to juggle with available information such as performing mental arithmetic; difficulty in shifting the focus from one topic to another, and defects in social cognition (e.g., reading people's reactions in social settings).

HOW TO GET COGNITIVE PROBLEMS ASSESSED?

There are three possible methods of identifying, assessing, and monitoring cognitive problems. These include periodical reviews by a psychiatrist, specialized testing by a psychologist, and diagnostic brain scans. Of these, regular monitoring in a clinical setting is often the only feasible option. Psychological testing to assess the cognitive problems in schizophrenia is a sophisticated procedure, and is not readily available everywhere. There are few psychologists who have the required training and expertise to perform such tests. Brain scanning techniques such as MRI hold the promise of precisely identifying and monitoring cognitive problems. But these techniques are still being developed, and are not easily accessible in all places.

WHAT CAN BE DONE ABOUT IMPAIRED COGNITIVE FUNCTIONS IN SCHIZOPHRENIA?

There are two ways of dealing with cognitive problems: treatment and prevention. Treatment strategies include the use of appropriate medications, maintaining an active daily routine, and participating in cognitive remedial therapy programs. Antipsychotic medications have been known to improve cognitive problems dramatically, especially during the early part of treatment. The newer antipsychotic medications (risperidone, olanzapine, quetiapine, ziprasidone and clozapine) seem to have an edge over the older generation of medications in producing a greater degree of improvement in negative symptoms and cognitive symptoms. It is also important to remember that using inappropriately higher doses of medication may actually worsen, instead of improving, certain aspects of cognition. Distinguishing frequently associated symptoms such as anxiety, depression or obsessions, and treating them with appropriate medications such as antidepressants, also makes a big difference in improving cognitive functioning.

Cognitive remedial therapy is a relatively new approach that is not widely available for routine use. This involves practicing various mental exercises, usually with the help of a computer. Other simple steps include the use of various memory aids (e.g., using a dosing box to take medications regularly, and a calendar to note down appointments), and generally maintaining an active structured routine.

Like many other things in life, the principle with cognition is use it or lose it.

In the small proportion of individuals who are prone to develop a progressive type of cognitive deterioration, prevention is more critical. Initiation of antipsychotic medications early, soon after the
first symptoms of illness appear, may have some value in limiting the deterioration in later years. Strict adherence to the recommended dose of medication over a period of time is also essential in lessening the degree of deterioration. Keeping symptoms under control and avoiding relapses of illness is perhaps the best approach to prevent cognitive deterioration. It is important to note that the indiscriminate use of recreational (street) drugs can worsen cognitive functions in vulnerable individuals.

CURRENT LIMITATIONS

While a lot has been learned from research over the past two decades, several questions still remain unanswered. First of all, it is not known if there are certain cognitive disturbances that are unique to schizophrenia. Cognitive problems of different sorts are seen in a number of other disorders such as Alzheimer's disease, and the type of difficulties that are specific to schizophrenia are yet to be clearly identified. Second, there is a continuing debate about the progression of cognitive problems: whether they get worse over a period of time or not. Third, there is a need to develop a method of identifying individuals who are more prone to develop cognitive problems than others. Having such a predictive strategy will help early recognition and possible prevention. Fourth, the areas of the brain that are involved in cognitive deficits need to be pin pointed. Lastly, there is a need to develop new treatment strategies. Cognitive deterioration is one aspect of schizophrenia for which we do not have an effective treatment strategy at present. Clozapine is, so far, the most effective treatment available to deal with cognitive problems; but it demands extra monitoring efforts from the clinic staff, clients, and the families.

RESEARCH IN PROGRESS

Cognitive aspects of schizophrenia have become the most active area of research in the past five years. Researchers are working on identifying the exact nature of cognitive problems experienced by people with schizophrenia, and have developed appropriate tests to measure and monitor them. Functional imaging has been another active area of research. Scanning devices such as the MRI and PET imaging are being used to study the brain mechanisms involved in causing cognitive problems. Also, major pharmaceutical companies are actively investing in the development and testing of newer medications that are likely to offer greater benefits in improving cognitive problems. Psychologists, occupational therapists, and specialists in education are involved in developing various cognitive remedial strategies that could be incorporated into day treatment programs and daily routine.

CONCLUSION
Our efforts to understand schizophrenia seem to unfold as if we were peeling the layers of an onion. At first it appeared that positive
symptoms were the only problem. Antipsychotic medications have been greatly helpful in controlling these symptoms. As these medications became widely available, the problem of negative symptoms became apparent. The new second generation antipsychotic drugs offer some hope that negative symptoms can also be conquered. Cognitive problems are the next ones to tackle in the ongoing battle with this devastating disorder. Solving them presents a significant challenge.
Understanding the origins of cognition and brain mechanisms is likely to help us not only in dealing with schizophrenia, but also in unravelling the mysteries surrounding other mental illnesses. ●

CHAPTER 13:Relapse And Chronic Illnesses

RELAPSE

The nature of schizophrenia is such that the positive symptoms (hallucinations, delusions, etc.) tend to reoccur. It is important, therefore, to be aware that the ill person is likely to experience a relapse, and to watch for the early warning signs that their condition is getting out of control again. The behaviours that indicate a relapse are usually the same as those that occurred prior to the first episode, for example:

- sleeplessness
- increased social withdrawal
- deterioration of personal hygiene
- thought and speech disorder
- signs of visual and auditory hallucinations (e.g., listening excessively to loud music, usually with headphones, perhaps in an attempt to drown out the voices).

Relapse can occur for a number of reasons, as well as for no apparent reason. Some potential clues are listed below

- Stopping medication for a long enough period of time that acute symptoms may reappear
- Insufficient dosage of medication to prevent the return of acute symptoms
- Lack of support, either at home or from community services
- Severe emotional stress, e.g., the death of a loved one, the loss of a job, the move to a new home
- Physical exhaustion
- Usage of alcohol or street drugs

Sometimes the cause may be something that can be dealt with quite easily. For example, medication can be increased, a brief hospital stay can be arranged, or more support can be found.

Health care professionals warn that relapse can occur during a period called self-cure. (This also occurs in other illnesses, such as diabetes and arthritis.) Usually, such an attempt occurs three to five years after a diagnosis of schizophrenia has been made. It is a time when the ill individuals, tired of the disease, decides to take matters into their own hands. They may stop taking prescribed medication, may join a cult, may try to exorcize the illness out of the body, may do strenuous exercise to get rid of it, may consume vast quantities of vitamins or herbal medicines, and so on.

A relapse is very disappointing, but is common among sufferers of various chronic diseases. Whether the ill person goes through a period of carelessness, forgetfulness, or rebelliousness, he/she is simply being human. Unfortunately, however, this makes a person with schizophrenia particularly vulnerable to relapse.

The best way to prevent relapses, and deal with them when they happen, is to plan ahead by developing strategies both for avoidance and occurrence. Discuss these plans with the ill individual while he/she is in a stable phase, and also with the attending physician(s). By knowing the illness, you and the person with schizophrenia can be prepared to watch for signs of relapse, and seek immediate medical attention when they appear. Try to establish an agreement with the ill individual that, for example, will deter him/her from stopping medication, or that will encourage him/her to advise you or the
doctor when the feeling of losing control returns. Assure the ill person that he/she will not be abandoned should a relapse occur, but also make it clear as to what behaviours will not be tolerated, e.g., extreme aggression or violence.

While every effort must be made to persuade people with schizophrenia to take their medication voluntarily, most provincial mental health laws provide some form of assisted community treatment. Where a person has a severe illness, has a history of not taking prescribed treatment, and has frequent relapses, he/she may be required by law to take treatment in the community (as opposed to a hospital environment). If he/she refuses to comply with the treatment order, then he/she may be involuntarily admitted to a hospital. This can be a very helpful measure to those (relatively few) families who experience this problem. For more information on assisted community treatment orders, consult your provincial Schizophrenia Society, and a mental health or legal professional with expertise in this area.

Awareness and readiness can help your family prevent or minimize relapses. A plan is your weapon in the battle against schizophrenia.

RISK OF SUICIDE

With schizophrenia the possibility of suicide is an ever-present fact. The illness involves depression, delusions, and sometimes command hallucinations that may tell the person to attempt suicide. There is a tendency to act impulsively. E. Fuller Torrey, notes in <u>Surviving Schizophrenia: A Family Manual</u> that an estimated ten percent of all people with schizophrenia kill themselves. As in the general population, men are more likely to complete suicide, while women attempt it more often. Suicide, when it happens, occurs most commonly during the first five years of illness. After this, the risk drops considerably.

Torrey suggests that "Those at highest risk have a remitting and lapsing course, good insight (e.g., they know they are sick), have a poor response to medication, are socially isolated, hopeless about the future, and have a gross discrepancy between their earlier achievements and their current level of function.

Sometimes a suicide is methodically planned and deliberately committed. At other times, a suicide may be accidental — that is, the victim is acting out an hallucination or delusion when in a psychotic state. In either of the above situations there are some preventive measures you can take, although you can never guard completely against the possibility of suicide.

Here is a list of behaviours that may indicate suicide is being contemplated:

• The ill person talks about suicide: what it would be like to die, how to go about it, or makes comments such as "When I'm gone...," and so on. He/she is concerned about having a will, and about the distribution of possessions. He/she may begin giving away treasured belongings

• The ill individual expresses feelings of worthlessness, for example, "I'm no good to anybody"

• They show signs of hopelessness about the future, making comments like, "What's the use?"

• The ill person is showing signs of hearing voices or seeing visions that may be instructing him/her to do something dangerous

All talk of suicide or self-harm must be taken seriously. It is not true that someone who talks about suicide rarely does it. If the ill person begins to talk about suicide, or inflict wounds — no matter how superficial — upon him/herself, it is vital that you reach his/her therapist immediately. If this isn't possible, take the ill person to the hospital where he/she was previously admitted, or to the nearest emergency department. In many communities, there is a suicide hotline available.

Often, when someone commits suicide, family members stop going to support group meetings. The relatives of suicide victims may believe that their presence is too depressing for other members of the group. Families in support groups urge these people to keep attending meetings. As one father stated: "When a relative develops schizophrenia, the support group becomes your family, because so often you lose family and friends. Now, when you've lost your relative, you need your new family more than ever."

If suicide is attempted, and you are the one who discovers the ill individual during the act or soon thereafter, the following steps should be taken:

• Phone 911 immediately. (If this service is not available in your area, call the emergency number of the nearest hospital.)

• If appropriate, and if you are fully trained, perform CPR (cardiopulmonary resuscitation)

• Phone someone to come and be with you, whether it is at the hospital as you wait for news, or at home to take care of you

• Although it is not likely, be prepared for the possibility that the hospital may not admit the ill person, even after a suicide attempt

• Get in contact with your local support group, if there is one, and let them know what has happened

• Do not try to handle the crisis alone

• Do not hesitate to contact other support groups that deal specifically with grief and bereavement

TREATMENT-RESISTANT (REFRACTORY) SCHIZOPHRENIA

WHAT IS TREATMENT-RESISTANT SCHIZOPHRENIA?

Schizophrenia is an illness characterized by onset relatively early in life, most frequently during late adolescence or early adulthood. Its course is variable. However, evidence indicates that as many as one-third of individuals treated with antipsychotic medications (at least the older ones) do quite poorly. These individuals are frequently referred to as having treatment-resistant or refractory forms of the illness.

At present, there are no specific tests or measures that allow us to distinguish who will respond well to treatment or who will do poorly. There are certain factors which seem to increase the risk of doing poorly (e.g., male, early onset) but these are by no means absolute predictors. Some individuals fail to show effective response even in the earliest stages of the illness, while others may only show treatment-resistance across time. Fortunately however, there are those who show a rapid and effective response.

EVALUATING TREATMENT-RESISTANT SCHIZOPHRENIA

In those who are not responding effectively to treatment, various factors must be considered. It is important to review the diagnosis because schizophrenia-like symptoms are seen in other conditions, and this may influence treatment. Antipsychotic medication remains the cornerstone of treatment in schizophrenia, and failing to take the medication can be associated with persistent symptoms that can mimic treatment-resistance (when in fact, it is more related to not taking the medication or noncompliance). There is variability in responses to antipsychotic medications, with individuals showing response to certain medications and not to others. For this reason, it is important to try various agents with people who have not responded to one or more medications. Other behaviours, such as substance abuse, can exacerbate or diminish symptom control, and this too can result in an individual appearing to be refractory to treatment.

DEFINING OUTCOME MEASURES

Not so long ago, it was common to evaluate response to treatment along a single dimension, e.g., dealing only with positive symptoms such as hallucinations and delusions. However, it is now more common to see schizophrenia defined as an illness that can affect a number of dimensions, and therefore have different outcome measures. For example, we now speak of different symptom clusters which include not only the positive symptoms, but negative symptoms (loss of energy, decreased motivation); cognitive symptoms (disorganization, difficulties with attention and concentration); affective symptoms (depression), and so on. Similarly, it is now more common to look at not only symptom outcome measures but functional outcome measures, that is how an individual is able to carry out the normal daily activities required of all of us.

With these numerous measures now being evaluated, the scope of treatment response, or conversely treatment-resistance, has broadened. More specifically, individuals may show improvement in some of these measures, while failing to show the same degree of change in others. In this sense, treatment resistance is not seen as a single entity any longer, but rather a multi-dimensional process.

A SYSTEMATIC APPROACH TO TREATMENT-RESISTANT SCHIZOPHRENIA

In order to optimize treatment outcome, it is absolutely essential that a systematic approach be taken to treatment. This includes ensuring that different antipsychotics have been tried, and that this has been done in a way that maximizes the chance of success, for example, adequate doses for a sufficient duration of time. There is currently evidence that the newer antipsychotics, as well as having fewer side effects that characterized the older compounds, may have a broader clinical effect as well e.g., they may effect more of these different clinical symptoms. Thus, it is recommended that if individuals have not done well on the conventional or older antipsychotics, trials with the newer compounds should be undertaken.

Among the newer antipsychotics, which include clozapine, risperidone, olanzapine, and quetiapine, there is evidence that clozapine seems to work best in those individuals who have truly proven resistant to treatment with other agents, both old and new. Unfortunately, clozapine is associated with a particular side effect that requires ongoing blood monitoring, and for this reason some individuals choose not to take it. However, it is generally recommended that all individuals who have not demonstrated a good response to other antipsychotics have a trial of clozapine at some point. As a rule, this trial is often left until various other antipsychotic agents have been tried because of the need for the ongoing blood monitoring.

Even with those who have tried clozapine, it is possible to see only a partial response. At that point, what are called augmentation strategies are frequently invoked in order to further improve response. This involves the addition of other medications, or even ECT, to the existing antipsychotic, once again in an effort to maximize clinical response.
Agents that might be used as augmentation strategies include antidepressants, mood stabilizers, benzodiazepines, and even other antipsychotic medications in combination.

In treating ill persons, including those who prove to be treatment-resistant, it is essential that the approach include more than just medication. To this end, the best response seems to occur in those individuals who receive medication in addition to nonpharmacological interventions such as psychoeducation programs regarding the illness, rehabilitation programs, and ongoing individual and social therapeutic interventions. This often involves the coordination of a number of different health care professionals, and seems most successful when the treatment team can work collaboratively with the individual and his or her social supports e.g., a spouse or other family members.

CONCLUSION

In general, there is a sense that treatments for schizophrenia are improving, particularly more recently. It is a clinical reality that at present there are individuals who remain resistant to existing therapies, but ongoing developments and improvements in treatment serve to hold hope even for this particular group.

With all these options available, it is crucial that ill persons be evaluated and re-evaluated by their physician(s) on a regular and timely basis. It is estimated that as many as forty percent of ill persons continue to be on medications that provide less than optimum results. Every effort should be made to bring these ill people to the best level of functioning possible, for example, trials of newer medications.

New drugs provide better opportunities than ever for better stability and functional recovery. At the time of publication, a new drug known as Zeldox or Ziprasidone is awaiting approval from Canadian authorities. It is, therefore, advisable to keep abreast of the most up-to-date developments in drug therapy. New medications bring new hope for all who experience schizophrenia.

PREVENTION OF RELAPSE

DEFINITION

Relapse in the older psychiatric literature was always synonymous with re-admission to hospital. Outcome studies used rates of re-admission (relapse) as measures of outcome even though for families, and frequently for patients, re-hospitalizations were good things in that they offered respite from constant worry, or a chance at a re-assessment or better treatment, or a roof over one's head and nutritious meals.

More recently, relapse means a change of score on a symptom scale. At the beginning of a treatment program, for instance, the ill person may be given a symptom questionnaire. As they improve the score changes (goes either up or down depending on the questionnaire). A relapse is subsequently defined as a certain percentage change back to the pre- treatment value. This is a useful and measurable definition, but it is not foolproof. The questionnaire may not include questions that address the behaviour that, to the family and caregivers, signals imminent worsening of the ill individual. For example, sleepless nights or sudden aggression may alert people who know the ill person well that something is changing, however, this change in behaviour may not be reflected in the questions asked or answers given in the questionnaire.

In the future, relapse may be defined with respect to function: losing a job for instance; losing a friend, or failing a class. Functioning is probably more important to families and to the ill person than symptoms.

For the purpose of the following section, relapse will simply mean general worsening as perceived by the family and caregivers.

HOW TO PREVENT RELAPSE

Tried and true ways to prevent relapse are the reduction of stress, the provision of structure, the modulation of stimulation, and the maintenance of support.

Reducing Stress

Reducing the chance of being overstressed is like reducing the chance of being infected. You try to avoid possible sources of stress (just as you would avoid people who sneeze); you try to develop habits that counter the effects of stress (just as you would regularly wash your hands); you try to fortify your defenses against stress (just as you would eat a healthy diet with lots of vitamins), and you try to immunize yourself against stress (just as you would get a flu shot).

Avoiding stress means working part-time rather than full time, having a room of your own you can go to during a family party, and avoiding people who make you tense. Good counter stress habits are getting lots of sleep, good food, exercise, having friends you can talk to, and avoiding alcohol, drugs, and nicotine. You can fortify your defenses against stress, for example, by discussing what people have said and how you reacted to their comments, as well as how you might have misunderstood them and how you could have reacted. Developing good defenses are important issues to discuss with a therapist.

Immunizing against stress means taking prescribed medications. Just like inoculations, they may hurt a little temporarily but what is gained far outstrips what might be suffered.

Providing Structure

While lots of sleep is good, lying in bed not sleeping is bad. It allows thoughts and worries to crowd out reality. A person with schizophrenia needs a tight schedule for every day. That does not mean running wildly around — rest periods can be built into the schedule. An appointment calendar serves as an organizer and memory tool; using it can also give the ill individual a sense of accomplishment at the end of each day.

Moderating Stimulation

While too many stimuli cause stress, too few may encourage apathy and boredom. The task of the family and caregivers is to modulate the stimulation just enough. This is not easy but comes with practice. The person with schizophrenia should be urged to be active, but not so much that it becomes overwhelming. Generally, activities that involve fewer people are easier. A walk around the block together could be a start.

Introducing something new now and again is good, but novelty is always stressful. It is important to establish a routine, then you can make slight variations on the routine, but not all at once.

Maintaining Support

This refers mainly to emotional support but may include financial support as well. No matter what the person with schizophrenia says or how he/she behaves, the family needs to maintain a supportive stance. This can be at a distance if necessary. Support does not necessarily mean closeness. It means that the ill person knows that the family is always there for him/her no matter what. Ideally, this is accompanied by encouragement, praise, recognition of even minor accomplishments, and optimism.

If you notice behavioural changes in the ill person that you suspect may coincide with the onset of a relapse, bring it to the attention of a member of the treatment team immediately. Remember, relapse is a natural phase of the illness. With strength, courage, and lots of support,

the ill person can recover again! ●

CHAPTER 14: Best Practices In Rehabilitation

In Chapter 7 we discussed psychosocial treatment for schizophrenia. By intervening with ill persons, significant improvements in their recovery and quality of life can be achieved. This proven philosophy has led to the development of renowned concepts and programs in rehabilitation. In this chapter, we describe in detail the most successful responses to the psychosocial needs of persons with schizophrenia.

CLUBHOUSES

Best Practice Example:

Fitzroy Centre Clubhouse
170 Fitzroy Street, Charlottetown, Prince Edward Island

Established by the Canadian Mental Health Association, P.E.I. Division in 1989, Fitzroy Centre has over 300 members (people who participate in the Centre's programs). The average daily attendance to the Clubhouse is 85 to 100 members. Fitzroy Centre was designed in accordance with the International Clubhouse Model. It provides an environment specifically geared to support people with mental health problems. The Clubhouse goal is to help people achieve or regain the confidence and skills necessary to lead productive and socially satisfying lives. Members are initially encouraged to participate in club programs with which they feel comfortable. As their confidence and abilities improve they are encouraged and supported in their efforts to learn skills that will help them to enter the work force. Social and recreational activities are provided to members during evening hours and on Saturdays. The Clubhouse is divided into three main units: Members Services Unit, Housing Unit, and Employment Unit.

Members Services Unit

The two main goals of this unit are to provide pre-vocational training opportunities and social recreation activities for members. By participating in the various activities in the unit, members can learn clerical skills such as filing or typing while working on the Clubhouse's weekly newsletter; research skills such as recording and reporting of information on member participation, attendance, and success stories; communication skills through reaching out to members who do not regularly attend the club; meal planning by working with the Centre's food services section; store clerk by working in the Clubhouse canteen or thrift store; telephone operating skills by working with the switchboard at the club, and housekeeping (vacuuming, dusting, cleaning) by helping to keep the club clean and beautified.

Members have the opportunity to participate in recreation activities during evenings and weekends, and get involved in planning special occasion events.

Housing Unit

The primary objective of this unit is to help members obtain as independent a housing situation as they can maintain. Clubhouse staff work with members to access and maintain decent and affordable housing that suits their individual needs and capabilities. Housing may be sought in the community, or within a Clubhouse home or apartment. Fitzroy Centre operates several housing projects:

•   Longworth House – a ten bedroom house that provides a home environment

•   Fitzroy Centre Apartment Complex – a seventeen unit apartment complex located next to the Clubhouse. The individual apartment units allow occupants to live independently, while at the same time accessing support they need to live on their own

•   181 Kent Street Apartments – an eight unit complex for members who require only occasional support to live independently; and

•   Rent Subsidy Apartment – 15 independent apartments located around the city. Occupant members are provided a rent subsidy that is geared to their income

The Housing Unit also provides education to members in daily living skills, for example, financial management and budgeting, medication regimes, etc. It also maintains the reception area for the club, giving members the opportunity to learn how to greet visitors and direct them to various areas of the club. The unit is also responsible for repairs to Clubhouse facilities and care of the grounds. Members can get involved in painting, minor plumbing, carpentry, and obtaining estimates for repairs that they can't do themselves. They can also learn gardening and lawn maintenance.

Employment Unit

The philosophy of the Clubhouse concept is that members and staff run the Clubhouse facility together, with the members being the driving force of the program. They work alongside staff doing all the various jobs of the Housing Unit and Member Services Unit. They learn the life skills required for their job in the outside world, such as dressing neatly, being punctual, and interacting with fellow employees. The objective of the Fitzroy Centre's employment unit is to assist members in their efforts to attain their highest potential in the areas of employment and education.

The supports and services provided by the unit include:

•   Employment and Education Counselling – wherein members receive the help they need to set vocational and educational goals

•   Life Skills Instruction – helps members learn and apply coping skills to better manage their life situations, and to overcome employment barriers that may be preventing them from working

•   Employment Skills Training – offers training programs that prepare members for entry or re-entry into the work force, and organized job finding clubs for the members

•   Transitional Employment Placement (TEP) – offers part-time entry- level jobs within the community. The employment unit arranges the placements, and members work in the positions for six to nine months. TEP provides members with the opportunity to develop their confidence and good working habits in the real world

•   Job Search and Marketing Supports – this service is also known as Job Finding Clubs, and is offered during peak hiring times. Participating members receive assistance in all aspects of job searching (e.g., resume preparation, applications, contacting employers, job interviews, and follow-up). The unit has a Job Board which includes information received daily from Human Resources and Development Canada, local newspapers, employers, and other sources. Members are also individually informed of available job opportunities. Another aspect of this service is advocacy Clubhouse staff advocate for employment opportunities, and go out into the community to educate employers on the Centre's programs and services

- Education and Literacy – provides learning tools for members such as literacy tutoring, and interactive computer programs in math, writing, autoskills, typing, and reading. This service also organizes educational activities such as library trips, spelling bees, museum tours, and guest speakers. Staff provide support to members to help them achieve their educational goals, and offer assistance with referrals to educational institutions

The diversity of the programs offered at Fitzroy Centre allows members to set and achieve their individual life goals. Studies have shown that people who are involved in a Clubhouse experience less frequency of relapse, and report an improvement in their quality of life.

Best Practice Example:

Potential Place1130-10th Avenue S.W., Calgary, Alberta

Also based on the International Clubhouse model, and accredited accordingly, Potential Place is Calgary's restorative environment for people struggling with severe and persistent mental illness. It is designed as a place of transition from institutionalization to independent living.

Potential Place's primary goal is to help people with mental illness attain or regain the self-esteem, confidence, and social skills necessary to lead vocationally productive and socially satisfying lives. Through Clubhouse activities (see description above), and advocacy in the community, Potential Place works to dispel the stereotype beliefs about the mentally ill and their place in the real world. The Clubhouse's core belief is that what people who have mental illness need is not isolation as full-time patients, but rather integration into the real world. They have a right to meaningful, gainful employment (or volunteer positions), decent housing, a supportive community, opportunities for education and recreation in their communities, and the chance to contribute to society to the best of their abilities.

Members of Potential Place are accepted with all of their strengths, weaknesses, talents, history, experience, likes, dislikes, hopes, fears, and dreams for the future. The process of rehabilitation involves a process of gradual acceptance into a community providing equality, respect, and opportunity. With this kind of support, Potential Place helps up to 117 members monthly to work and become fully participating members of the community.

WOMEN'S MENTAL REHABILITATION PROGRAMS

In Chapter 8 we discussed the special needs and issues of women with schizophrenia. Women with the disorder tend to recover their ability to be socially active, and as such face the challenges of dating, sex, marriage, family planning, and having children all while dealing with schizophrenia. Rehabilitation programs designed to address the specific needs of females provide valuable education and support to women. Our Best Practice example of such a program is located in Toronto. Since 1995, the Clarke Institute Centre for Addiction and Mental Health has provided a program especially for women with schizophrenia. The service is comprised of:

- Comprehensive patient and family assessment
- Recommendations to treating clinicians
- Drug and psychosocial treatment
- Patient management during pregnancy and early parenthood
- Substance abuse counselling
- Sex education
- Parent training
- Relationship focus groups
- Self protection to avoid victimization
- Home based outreach programs

and has established linkages with community clinicians, agencies, and facilities in order that ill people have access to:

- Pediatricians
- Gynecologists
- Fitness programs
- Leisure activities
- Children's aid and protection services

As well, ill individuals have access to the Centre's many services for persons with schizophrenia, including:

- Stress-reduction focus groups
- Work-readiness programs

- Initial episode programs
- Family programs
- Psychoeducation
- Leisure groups

The program is staffed by two psychiatrists, a rotation of psychiatric residents from various countries, student doctors, two nurses, a social worker, and an occupational therapist. A variety of diverse cultures are represented on staff, offering knowledge and understanding of multicultural issues to the patients.

The clinic gets deeply involved in the special issues women with schizophrenia face. When the program is not equipped to deal with a matter, staff ensures the ill person is put in touch with an appropriate agency. For example, pregnant women and new mothers receive medical and counselling services from the program, including care in their own homes. When other help is required, such as baby clothing, or child welfare services, the clinic connects the mother with workers from other organizations. It also oversees care for mother and child by providing integrated services that encourage activities for mother and child such as fitness, drop-in centres, swimming or dancing lessons, and craft activities. Regular care by a pediatrician is also monitored by the clinic.

It is particularly interesting to note that this program for women with schizophrenia upholds the role of the family and other caregivers by maintaining close liaisons with them. As well, where children are involved, the clinic stays in contact with grandparents and other appropriate relatives, schoolteachers, and child welfare workers if applicable.
Overall, the program promotes and supports a network of friends and helpers for their patients. It recognizes the need for drug therapy, psychosocial treatment, and maintenance of general health. The service does its utmost to ensure the patients are socially active, and well instructed on issues surrounding sexual activity. Patients are monitored closely for depression and risk of suicide. The clinic also provides active and immediate outreach at times of crisis.

For a listing of women's rehabilitation programs in your area, we suggest you contact your local Schizophrenia Society chapter, or regional branch of the Canadian Mental Health Association.

ASSERTIVE COMMUNITY TREATMENT TEAMS (ACT)
(ALSO KNOWN AS THE CASE MANAGEMENT APPROACH)

Best Practice Example:

Douglas Hospital, 6875, boul. LaSalle
Verdun, Quebec H4H 1R3 Tel: 514-761-6131 ext. 2270

(there are many ACT teams across the province of Quebec and in several other provinces in Canada).

In the aftermath of de-hospitalization, provincial health ministries across Canada have pursued various initiatives to support individuals suffering from severe mental illness. A best practice result is found in the ACT approach to recovery. It facilitates adjustment to the illness, offering the ill person intensive individual support and case management.

In 1997, the Clarke Institute of Psychiatry published its research evidence on Best Practices in Mental Health Reform. The discussion paper states that "...ACT programs are superior for improving clinical status and reducing hospitalization." It also revealed that "...assertive community treatment is effective for very difficult-to-house populations such as the homeless." The paper found that ACT is the most comprehensive system of integrated care because it combines crisis intervention, treatment, and individual support. It is most suitable to severe sufferers requiring substantial care intervention.

ACT: HOW IT OPERATES

ACT is designed as an alternative to hospitalization for persons suffering from a severe and persistent mental illness such as schizophrenia. It provides round-the-clock continuous care and service in the community environment. The team directly treats,
rehabilitates, and supports its clients within a planned, coordinated, and efficient case management process.

The team typically consists of a case manager, clinical supervisor, program psychiatrist, program assistant, team coordinator, other multidisciplinary staff, and the client. On the day the ill individual is admitted to the program, he/she will be evaluated for his/her mental health status, treatment requirements, and practical needs for housing and finances. A plan is devised to guide the team until a comprehensive assessment and treatment plan is prepared

The comprehensive assessment will determine the client's mental and functional status and corresponding requirements. An individual
treatment plan is created for the client from the results of this evaluation. The client will be monitored for side effects and beneficial results of psychotropic medication. Supportive therapy is given to clients on an individual basis, and consists of discussions to help them understand and identify symptoms, lessen distress and symptomatology, improve role functioning, and increase participation in and satisfaction with treatment and rehabilitative services. A staff member who has experienced mental illness provides peer support.

The treatment plan involves the client's family, and promotes achievement of goals as chosen by the client. The plan is reviewed to establish client progress, and delineate his/her functional strengths and limitations. It is then revised in accordance with results. The goals and objectives of a treatment plan are regularly assessed, and the client's schedule of services is developed on a weekly basis.

ACT or Case Management teams are available in many communities across Canada. Contact your local hospital or mental health clinic for more information.

SIM PROGRAM (SUIVI INTENSIF DANS LE MILIEU)

This program was developed by the Louis H. Lafontaine Hospital in Quebec. Loosely translated, SIM means intensive follow-up care in the community. The program is based on the same philosophy as ACT.
A SIM program gives people with schizophrenia support in different aspects of their lives that they find problematic. The support can be provided on a daily basis or a weekly basis, according to the needs of the ill person. This intervention is performed in the ill individual's home by a specially trained health professional or a nurse. The SIM caregiver helps the ill person get reacquainted with the tasks of day- to-day living, and finds a means of overcoming any obstacles the ill person encounters in daily life. The primary objective of SIM is to enable people with

schizophrenia to establish an independent lifestyle.

On the whole, this treatment helps to improve the state of health of the ill person, while decreasing the risk of relapse. The SIM caregiver is available to answer any questions the ill person has concerning medication and/or symptoms associated with the disorder. The caregiver makes sure that the ill person is taking his/her medication as prescribed and is following the treatment plan. The patient is also monitored for side effects. Stress factors in the ill individual's life are identified, along with the means of overcoming or reducing them. The SIM caregiver also acts as a liaison between the ill person and his/her treatment team.

SIM's goal is to give the ill person the tools required for independent living, and the extra help he/she needs in areas that give the individual particular difficulty as a result of the illness. A SIM caregiver will provide guidance and/or hands-on help in such areas as: preparation of meals, finances and budgeting, finding housing, and gaining familiarity with community resources and activities that are available to the ill person. Where needed, he/she will accompany the ill person to the grocery store for shopping, and on public transportation for appointments or activities.

The SIM caregiver also supports the social rehabilitation of the ill person, helping him/her to re-integrate comfortably into his/her previous activities, or find new interests that are suitable.

For a listing of follow-up care programs in your area, we suggest you contact your local Schizophrenia Society chapter, or regional branch of the Canadian Mental Health Association.

CRISIS RESPONSE SYSTEMS (CRS)

Best Practice Example:

Manitoba provides extensive community-based emergency and crisis services to people who have formerly accessed institutional services, and are a threat to themselves or others. Crisis situations may arise from recurrent episodes of psychosis, poverty, homelessness, unemployment, or loss of support services. Hospitalization may not be the most effective approach to manage the ill person's crisis.

The Youth Emergency Crisis Stabilization System is one example of Manitoba's crisis response services. It is specifically targeted to children, adolescents, and their families and caregivers who are
experiencing psychosocial and related emergencies, providing them help in a timely and appropriate fashion. Access to this service is through a 24 hour/7 days per week intake and triage system. Crises are then referred to the Mobile Crisis Team, and non-crises are referred to the appropriate service.

The Mobile Crisis Team (MCT) will stabilize the crisis, provide on-site services, and develop treatment strategies for ongoing intervention.

The team includes a Clinical Follow-up Facilitator who will assist clients to access the services they need in order to carry out the intervention strategies developed by the Mobile Crisis Team. The MCT may refer the client to a Brief Treatment Team (BTT) who responds to the client within one day. The BTT is a multidisciplinary team who provides time-limited, solution focused treatment to clients, addressing issues and events that lead up to the crisis.

The MCT may also refer a client to a Crisis Stabilization Unit (there is one location for girls, and another for boys). These units are for clients who are in extreme distress, and may need a few days to reintegrate into their environment following their crisis. The MCT also offers Home Based Crisis Intervention Services to help clients and their families get back to a functioning level after experiencing a crisis. These services are provided immediately, and include support and homemaker services. As well, the MCT may help to facilitate reconnections with educational services or schools following a crisis situation.

Generally speaking, crisis response systems offer a range of integrated

caregiver's residence. The goal of the program is to provide respite care services to the ill person in his/her own home environment whenever possible.

This program is currently offered in the following British Columbia health regions: Vancouver/Richmond, North Shore, Fraser Valley, South Fraser, Simon Fraser, and Coast Garibaldi. For more information, contact the British Columbia Schizophrenia Society at 604-270-7841.

Best Practice Example:

Seneca House

Seneca House is a charitable organization funded by the Winnipeg Regional Health Authority. It is a place where adults with mental illness can go when they are experiencing emotional difficulties. The philosophy of Seneca House is that people who have experienced a mental health problem are best able to provide empathy and support to others in similar situations. All staff members have personal experience with mental illness. With their help, guests of Seneca House learn to cope with their distress.

Seneca House provides opportunities for respite and peer support through short-term residential stays of up to five nights (once per calendar month to a maximum of seven times per year) in a safe and comfortable home environment. Guests may use this time to explore their feelings, attitudes, beliefs, challenges, and choices, and to learn about other community resources that can assist them in their recovery process. Seneca House provides round the clock trained staff, six private bedrooms that include a secure box for medication and valuables, meals, and laundry facilities – all at no cost to the client. It is open twenty-four hours a day, seven days a week.

Access to this service is (usually) through referral from a health service provider. The service is targeted to people who have used nmental health services. Guests must be able to make a commitment to: refrain from harm or violence to self or others; to be abstinent from alcohol or street drugs during their stay; to administer their own medication without supervision; to attend to daily living tasks without assistance (or with assistance from an attendant who will accompany them to the home), and to respect the rights and needs of their fellow guests.

Staff at Seneca House are Peer Support Workers with training and experience in crisis intervention and suicide prevention. Using their personal experience with mental illness and recovery, they strive to address the self-identified needs of each guest.

Seneca House provides employment opportunities to people with mental illness who are ready and able to assist others with the

recovery process. Potential staff candidates must have a grade 12 High School Diploma or equivalent, CPR and First Aid Certification (or the ability to obtain same in 3 months), and Non-Violent Crisis Intervention certification (or the ability to obtain same in 3 months).

To find out if there are respite or peer support programs in your area, we suggest you contact your local Schizophrenia Society chapter, or regional branch of the Canadian Mental

Health Association. ●

CHAPTER 15: Multiculturalism & Schizophrenia

ISOLATION

SSC recognizes the additional challenges and difficulties imposed upon some families from ethnically diverse backgrounds. They may be isolated from mainstream Canadian social support systems and health care systems. The key reasons for this are:

•   Language barriers which interfere with assessment and treatment of ill people

•   In some cultures, schizophrenia is viewed as a punishment of the ill person — the stigma associated with it is therefore formidable, and families and ill individuals may try to hide in shame from the disease

•   A reliance on family members to deal with the illness

•   A lack of sensitivity and awareness by professionals in diagnosing and treating people with schizophrenia from different cultures

•   A lack of collaboration between community organizations, agencies, and institutions to increase accessibility to treatment

•   A lack of ability, particularly for new immigrants, to pay for psychological or psychiatric services

Culture influences how people with schizophrenia and their families respond to the disorder. Some immigrant Canadians suffering from schizophrenia may try to ignore the illness; accept it as fate, or seek advice from a religious leader. The afflicted person is not likely to seek treatment from a physician about mental and emotional problems. In some cultures, it is unacceptable to complain to a health professional about feelings such as despondency, loneliness, or the desire to die. It is more probable that physical symptoms such as sleeplessness, change in appetite, or weight loss will be relayed. In other words, some immigrant people with schizophrenia may translate their emotions into physical ailments when talking to a physician.

THE NEED FOR AWARENESS AND EDUCATION

Outreach to multicultural groups is required to promote an awareness and understanding of schizophrenia. There is, at times, a lack of knowledge about the disorder and how it can be recognized; about our mental health care system and how it can treat schizophrenia, and about how to gain access to drug therapy and psychotherapy.

SSC, and the contributing families, have identified areas where work is needed to support Canadians from diverse cultures to understand schizophrenia, and get proper treatment for ill individuals. They include:

• Translation of information and educational materials into various languages, so as to support multicultural families' access to knowledge

• Work with ethnic press, radio and TV stations to promote awareness of schizophrenia

• Dissemination of materials on schizophrenia through immigrant service agencies and ethnic community associations

• Increased coordination and joint efforts among community and mental health organizations that serve the multicultural community;

• Gathering and dissemination of research data pertaining to various ethnicity response levels to drug therapies amongst the medical professions

• Promotion of awareness of the different values diverse cultures hold, which impact their attitudes toward mental illness, amongst health caregivers

• Invitation of members of ethno-specific communities as guest speakers to meetings of support groups and associations involved in helping those who suffer from schizophrenia

• Development of culture brokers (persons who help to bridge the gap between the ill person's culture and that of the health caregivers by translating professional jargon and attitudes to ill people and his/her families, and by helping the professionals understand how the ill person's culture impacts their problems)
and promotion of their involvement with schizophrenia organizations

• Advocacy in the area of ethno-specific housing, social support, and employment programs, and integration of mental health services and immigration services, and

• Work with colleges, universities, and professional accreditation bodies to encourage the adoption of culturally sensitive training in the curriculum for health caregivers

Some key points:

• Immigration does not cause schizophrenia; however, the stress surrounding it can compound the problem

• A physician cannot accurately diagnose the ill individual unless the emotional symptoms the person has experienced are revealed, along with the physical ones

• It is incumbent upon you to help the ill person by making physicians and health caregivers aware of your family's attitudes toward mental illness

• Although schizophrenia does not differentiate between races and cultures, drug treatment may affect some cultures differently than others

• Be sure to use all the federal and provincial government services, and ethno-specific community association programs available to you. They may be able to provide interpreters and other assistance you require to get diagnosis and treatment for the ill individual

• All of the other chapters in this book may also be of help to you. Please read them carefully to help you understand schizophrenia, and how it impacts you and the ill person in your family, and

• You are welcome at SSC and its affiliate organizations: please let us help you!

HELP FOR FAMILIES

CULTURAL INTERPRETATION SERVICES (CIS)

Hospitals and health care facilities across Canada are becoming more aware of their responsibility to provide interpretation services for patients who are not proficient in English or French. It is becoming widely recognized that language barriers result in poor quality care, which adds to the burden of costs to the health care system.

Research has proven that clear and understandable communication between health professionals and patients leads to better results.

An example of a CIS service can be found at the Centre for Addiction and Mental Health in Toronto. The Centre provides this service to patients/families who have specific language and/or translation requirements. A trained interpreter is available for clinical visits to ensure the ill individual's concerns are understood, thereby enabling the treatment process. The CIS also works to help the Centre identify areas of service that are not sensitive to race, culture, ethnicity, gender, age, abilities, religion, and sexual orientation, and develop strategies to address these gaps in service.

The role of an interpreter in a clinical setting is to:

•   Ensure the patient understands his/her rights with respect to treatment

•   Provide accurate interpretation of the meaning and content of information given by the patient

•   Facilitate communication between the patient and clinician

•   Respect the integrity and right to confidentiality of all parties involved

•   Try to establish a rapport with the patient

•   Avoid situations where there may be a conflict of interest

•   Reveal and correct errors in communication or misunderstandings that occur

•   Respect the families they help by not interfering with conversations between patients and family members

Often a CIS service can be accessed through the Special Services department of the hospital or clinic you are attending. Please be sure to ask if interpreters are available at your health facility, or if provisions for this type of service have been established within your community.
Where available, make arrangements to have an interpreter accompany you on clinical visits. The better you are understood, the better able the health care system is to treat you appropriately and effectively. ●

CHAPTER 16: Stigma – Misunderstanding Schizophrenia

PUBLIC PERCEPTION

"One thing I find really hard about my illness is the stigma."

– Shawna, a person with schizophrenia.

What is the biggest problem people who have been treated for mental illness face when trying to resume a normal life? Most will say it is simply that others do not accept them. They have difficulty in finding friends, housing, and work. They feel the sting of discrimination in almost everything they attempt. Many times people with this disorder feel that even old friends and family are uncomfortable in their presence. Overall, they experience a feeling of being cut off from society. The stigma that still surrounds mental illness can sometimes be the most disabling component of schizophrenia.

Public perception of mental illness is partly driven by fear: fear of disease, fear of the unknown, and fear of violence. When people do not understand, they often make wild guesses. Some cultures believe mental illness is the work of evil spirits, while other cultures feel bad blood, poisons, or a lack of moral integrity causes it. As we learn more about the biological causes of mental illness, many of these wrong beliefs will, hopefully, fade.

Better health education programs can help to correct these myths and misunderstandings. Providing psychiatric treatment in general hospitals rather than in mental hospitals, and keeping recovering individuals in their own communities with the necessary supports, will also help to overcome the prejudice against mentally ill persons.

The devastating reality of the public's wrong perception is its impact on those that suffer from the disease, along with their families. Stigma has caused families to shy away from public involvement for fear of creating further hurt or embarrassment for the ill person and other family members. As a result of these years of silence about the illness, the general public sees no evidence of an unmet need. Without powerful advocates and government recognition and support, funds necessary to carry research forward have fallen far behind those of other illnesses.

MYTHS ABOUT VIOLENCE AND SPLIT PERSONALITY

Schizophrenia is one of the most misunderstood disorders of our day. A common myth about mental illness is based on the Hollywood portrayal of a mad person. The public has impressions of mentally ill people being institutionalized behind locked doors and barred windows; being physically restrained by cuffs or straight jackets; and being committed by the courts due to their behaviour. There is a common fear that mentally ill persons are dangerous, unpredictable, and aggressive. The myth of danger is perpetuated by 1) the public's lack of knowledge and 2) the media. Television and movie dramas frequently portray mentally ill persons as violent, homicidal objects
of dread. Newspapers and magazines also exaggerate events where mental disorders are involved.

The truth is that mentally and emotionally disturbed persons are usually anxious, fearful of others, and passive. There are situations in which mentally ill persons may become violent and aggressive, such as if they are acting out as a result of a delusion or hallucination. The good news is that when they are properly treated with antipsychotic medication, this aggression and violence will go away.

The second common misconception about schizophrenia comes from the notion that, by definition, it means having a split personality.
Schizophrenia is not a splitting of the personality into multiple parts, not a Jekyll and Hyde phenomenon, despite the popular hold of the Robert Louis Stevenson story. Most people with chronic schizophrenia are much too ill to carry off double lives. Split personalities are rare and are a form of hysteria, not schizophrenia. Nevertheless, the idea that schizophrenia equals split personality is pervasive. When people in everyday life describe something as schizophrenic, they mean split into two separate parts. How did the confusion start?
In 1911, the psychiatrist Eugen Bleuler invented the term schizophrenia to

describe the disorder. (Schizophrenia comes from the Greek schizo meaning split, and phrenia which means mind.) What Bleuler was trying to convey by the term was the split between perception and reality. Today many psychiatrists regret the existence of the term because it is misunderstood.

Misunderstanding can cause serious and unnecessary grief. It is important that we all take responsibility for sharing our knowledge about schizophrenia with others: for their sake, for our sake, and most

importantly, for the sake of those who have this disorder! ●

CHAPTER 17: Research - The Hope For A Cure

LATEST DEVELOPMENTS

TECHNOLOGY

We are in the midst of a knowledge explosion about brain chemistry. Research indicates that schizophrenia is not a psychological weakness, nor is it caused by parenting. It is a physical disorder: EEG's (electroencephalograms) show that the electrical impulses used by the brain to send messages to other parts of the body are abnormal in many people with schizophrenia. Chemical research shows chemical abnormalities of proteins and neurotransmitters in the brain of many people with schizophrenia. For example, some people have been found to have an excess of dopamine (neuro-transmitter) while others do not have sufficient amounts. With devices such as CT (computerized tomography) and MRI scans (magnetic resonance imaging), scientists have been able to take pictures of the brain. These imaging tools show that the brain structure of some people with schizophrenia is different from people without the illness. About one- third of people with schizophrenia have enlarged ventricles (small spaces in the brain through which cerebral spinal fluid circulates).

MRI scan research has produced some exciting results in the recent past. In November 2000, the Institute of Psychiatry in London, England reported results of a brain imaging study. Findings suggest substantial brain changes are evident at the earliest stages of schizophrenia, even before the appearance of positive symptoms. MRI scans revealed differences in the structure of key regions of the brain (such as the temporal lobe) for people experiencing psychosis. All
participants in the study had suffered symptoms of psychosis for three months or less, and some had never taken antipsychotic medication. Thus the difference in brain structure exists at least as early as the prodromal stage (before detection, or in the very early stages of the illness) of the disorder. Brain imaging may, therefore, help identify early warning signs of the illness.

PET (positron emission tomography) scans also show that the brains of people with schizophrenia function or work differently. Very often, there is decreased blood flow to the frontal lobes as well as decreased glucose utilization in the same area. The CT and MRI scans show the structure of the brain, while PET scans show brain functioning patterns. Active parts of the brain use more glucose, so PET scans taken after injections of glucose tagged with radioactive atoms can show which parts of the brain are being used during different activities. For example, when the person looks at a picture, the glucose instantly concentrates in the visual cortex at the back of the head.

Dr. Philip Seeman, a scientist at the University of Toronto explains:

"CT and MRI tell you whether the building structure is there, but PET tells you if there are any people in there, if they are having a party or what they are doing… It can truly give you the picture of a thought rather than the anatomy of the brain. It's perhaps five times more expensive than CT or MRI, but PET is a major tool."

PET scanners exist at medical research centres in Hamilton, Vancouver, Montreal, and Toronto, and may eventually be available in other larger urban centres in Canada.

Dr. Sandy McEwan, nuclear medicine physician at the Cross Cancer Institute in Edmonton describes an imaging device called a SPECT (single photon emission computed tomography) scanner as the "poor man's PET". Using this scanner and a radioactive compound (HMPAO), it is possible to measure blood flow in the same manner as a PET scanner, but at significantly less cost. The results of SPECT studies also show reduced blood flow in frontal lobes of people with schizophrenia.

Dr. McEwan foresees that this test may well become a routine procedure in the future. Many large hospitals throughout Alberta already have SPECT scanners.

At last, it seems beyond dispute that the hallucinations, delusions, paranoid thinking, and bizarre behaviour typical of schizophrenia result from an organic abnormality in the brain, as first reported by a team of scientists at the University of Toronto, led by Dr. Philip Seeman.

Dr. Seeman reported in 1977 that post mortem study of the brains of people who had suffered from schizophrenia showed an abnormally

large number of dopamine receptors in three tiny central areas of the brain. Since that discovery, research continues to provide evidence that schizophrenia is a physical disorder of the brain.

GENETICS

There are strong indications that there are genetic factors involved in developing schizophrenia. Three key pieces of evidence (listed below) support genetic factors as the primary causes of schizophrenia.

THE GENETIC LINK TO SCHIZOPHRENIA

1.   The risk for schizophrenia is greater for an identical twin of an individual with schizophrenia (identical twins have almost 100% of their genetic make-up in common), than for a fraternal twin of an individual with schizophrenia (fraternal twins have about 50% of their genetic make-up in common)

2.   The risk for schizophrenia is greater for close relatives of an individual with schizophrenia than for individuals in the general population who do not have a close relative with schizophrenia

3.   The risk for schizophrenia is greater for biological relatives of an individual with schizophrenia than for adoptive relatives

Genetic counselling is an important part of health care that should be available for all individuals with schizophrenia and their immediate relatives. Currently, genetic counselling for schizophrenia can provide information on estimated risks for developing the illness in close relatives of an individual with schizophrenia. In the future, genetic testing (which is currently unavailable) may be able to help with the diagnosis of people who are at risk for developing the disorder of genetic subtypes of schizophrenia. The main purpose of genetic research, however, is to understand the underlying mechanism of schizophrenia so that better and more specific treatments may be developed.

A study that scanned DNA from all 23 chromosomes from twenty- two large Canadian families (approximately three hundred individuals) with a

strong family history of schizophrenia (or related illnesses) has indicated where some genes for schizophrenia may reside. With the help of these families, researchers at the Clinical Genetics Research Program (CAMH/University of Toronto), headed by Dr.
Anne Bassett, and in collaboration with a U.S. group at Rutgers University, have found evidence that genes responsible for creating a predisposition for developing schizophrenia are likely to be found on chromosomes 1 and 13.

The finding on chromosome 1, in particular, promises to lead to the identification of a susceptibility gene for schizophrenia. The search for the specific gene, however, is not easy, since there are hundreds of genes in these chromosomal areas. It is like looking for a faulty brick (a specific genetic change) in a house (the gene) on a street in a city of a large country (the chromosome), but starting from the whole world (the entire human genome). The neighbourhood (chromosomal region) has been narrowed down for one of these houses (genes) to a certain region on chromosome 1. And there is another city-sized region on chromosome 13.

Genetic models (theories that attempt to predict the inheritance patterns of illnesses) suggest that schizophrenia may be caused by the interactive effect of several genes. The fact that there are significant linkage findings to two different chromosomes (1 and 13) in the same set of Canadian families with schizophrenia supports the likelihood of multiple genetic causes even in inherited forms of schizophrenia.

Schizophrenia is a complex illness. There are other genes on other chromosomes, as well as non-genetic factors, that probably play a part in the development of schizophrenia. In other words, it is not possible to simply look at a person's DNA and tell if there is an increased risk for schizophrenia. While there is much work ahead to identify, and learn about, the genes and non-genetic factors that contribute to the disorder, the success of this recent finding is very encouraging.

Another exciting finding is the discovery of a genetic syndrome known as 22q Deletion Syndrome (22qDS). It is associated with a chromosomal abnormality, and occurs in approximately one in two thousand to one in four thousand births. This means 22qDS is more common than other conditions like Huntington's disease and Duchenne muscular dystrophy. Approximately twenty-five percent of individuals with 22qDS develop schizophrenia, and up to two percent of individuals with schizophrenia may have 22qDS, indicating that 22qDS represents a genetic subtype of schizophrenia. The clinical signs and symptoms, structural brain findings, and cognitive profile of 22qDS-schizophrenia are all similar to those in other forms of schizophrenia. What is different is that people with a 22qDS subtype of schizophrenia have physical features and learning difficulties associated with the genetic syndrome.

It is interesting to note that approximately ninety percent of 22qDS cases are sporadic. In other words, this genetic form of schizophrenia usually presents itself in an individual whose family has no history of the illness. The mechanism of how and why this sporadic deletion occurs is not known, but we do know that it is nothing the parents did or did not do that caused the deletion. It is a chance occurrence. In the other ten percent of cases, one of the parents has 22qDS and has passed it on to their child. Because the physical findings associated with 22qDS can be quite subtle and vary from one person to the next, often a parent does not know that they have 22qDS until their child is diagnosed.

22qDS, which is also known as velocardiofacial syndrome or DiGeorge syndrome, usually has several other associated features, which can include: learning difficulties, speech or palate problems, characteristic but subtle facial features, congenital heart and other birth defects, hypocalcemia (low calcium levels in the blood), and thrombocytopenia (low platelet levels in the blood). Because the physical features are often subtle and the condition is not yet well known, 22qDS is under-recognized, especially in adults. Clinical screening criteria to help doctors and other clinicians better recognize 22qDS are now available. 22qDS may be definitively diagnosed using specialized chromosomal testing called Fluorescence In-Situ Hybridization (FISH), a special test that is usually ordered by a medical geneticist or other specialist with expertise in recognizing people with 22qDS. The ability to diagnose the syndrome is beneficial for both prevention and early detection of treatable illnesses, as well as genetic counselling.

There are important treatable illnesses associated with 22qDS that may develop at any age, and that doctors can monitor through simple blood tests. While there are no blood tests for psychiatric illnesses, an individual known to have 22qDS can be monitored for changes in behaviour and mood (possible indicators of schizophrenia). If changes develop, the person may benefit from early detection of the illness in the prodromal stage (before detection, or in the very early stages of the illness), allowing for immediate treatment and better chances of recovery. For individuals with a 22qDS subtype of schizophrenia, monitoring for onset of hypocalcemia (which can cause seizures) or thyroid abnormalities, both treatable conditions, is important.

RECOVERY

REHABILITATION

"Myth: Rehabilitation can be provided only after stabilization.

Reality: Rehabilitation should begin on Day One. "

Dr. Courtenay Harding, University of Colorado School of Medicine

Some of the most recent and hopeful news in schizophrenia research is emerging from studies in the field of psychosocial rehabilitation.

New studies challenge several long-held myths in psychiatry about the inability of people with schizophrenia to recover from their illness. It now appears that such myths, by maintaining an overall pessimism about outcomes, may significantly reduce ill people's opportunities for improvement and/or recovery. In fact, the long-term perspective on schizophrenia should give everyone a renewed sense of hope and optimism. Clinicians who investigate the long-term course and prognosis (a forecast of the course of the disorder) of schizophrenia are now presenting a very different picture of the illness from the gloomy scenario painted just a few years ago. Rehabilitation programs have evolved dramatically to improve the quality of life and functional recovery of people with schizophrenia. New and better drug therapies continue to be produced. Also, studies show that schizophrenia is not a disorder that progresses with age. The longer a person is free from acute episodes, the better the chances for a full recovery. The importance of family input for treatment, and the benefits of good relationships between clinicians and families, are now well established. Families need and want education, information, coping and communication skills, emotional support, and to be treated as collaborators. For this reason, knowledgeable clinicians will make a special effort to solicit involvement of family members and caregivers. Clinicians, individuals with the disorder, and families should work together to identify needs and appropriate interventions to help the ill person. Everyone involved should be able to have realistic yet optimistic expectations about improvement and possible recovery.

TREATMENT STRATEGIES

Schizophrenia is a long-term disorder. According to research, the first few years of the illness may determine the outcome. In other words, it is very likely that the success of interventions in the first years following onset will significantly impact whether the ill person has a good recovery, or suffers from chronic relapses. Furthermore, the time between onset of psychosis and effective treatment is, according to contemporary thinking, a significant factor in recovery. Young people who experience prolonged psychotic symptoms are at risk of actually suffering further neurobiological deficits, along with vocational, educational, and psychosocial delays.

The result of these findings, coupled with the influence of leading-edge programs such as the Early Psychosis Prevention and Intervention Centre (EPPIC) in Australia (see Chapter 5, Early Intervention), has made early intervention the current focus of research for treatment strategies. There are several early intervention programs across Canada. They are similar in approach and scope. The Calgary Early Psychosis Treatment and Prevention Program (EPP), for example, uses a case-management approach to treatment, offering its clients case management, psychiatric management and medication strategies, cognitive-behaviour therapy, group therapy, and family interventions. Family intervention programs are representative of a new concept in psychoeducational intervention, and have achieved worldwide recognition. Research has shown that these programs, when combined with medication, are far superior to medication strategies alone in reducing relapses. Furthermore, studies have determined that the issues and challenges confronting a family of a person with schizophrenia are different according to the stage of the illness. Also, newly diagnosed individuals and their relatives may be more responsive to a family program tailored to their individual needs as opposed to a group program. The course of schizophrenia can be broken into four key stages:

FOUR STAGES OF COPING WITH SCHIZOPHRENIA

1)   Before Detection – the early or prodromal phase

2)   After Detection Grief and Stress – beginning treatment

3)   Towards Recovery, Coping, Competence, and Adaptive Functioning – recovery process

4)   First Relapse and Prolonged Recovery – acute episode and long-term prognosis

In the first stage families are faced with the shock and upheaval caused by the behavioural changes in their ill family member. They need to access appropriate treatment, as well as obtain information about what the individual is experiencing. At this point, it is important that families receive counselling on the early warning signs of schizophrenia and related disorders, where to get help, and how to minimize disruption within the family unit, and reduce stress in the ill person's day-to-day life. (This is important because a firm diagnosis may take up to one year. In the interim, the ill person needs medical attention, and the family needs information.)

In the second stage, families must deal with the diagnosis of schizophrenia, and the beginning of treatment. They need comprehensive information about the disorder, and about their role in the recovery process. They may also need some help dealing with their emotions and the distress caused by the diagnosis.

In the third stage, families need to learn how to cope with the stress imposed upon them as they help their ill family member through the recovery process. They may need professional resources to assist in some areas, and to offer coping strategies. Families require information during this phase about the treatments the ill individual is undergoing, about the appropriate level of care as recovery progresses, and about early warning signs of relapse.

In the fourth stage, families may need to review their understanding of psychosis. The ill person will need treatment for an acute episode, and the family will need to understand the long-term prognosis. More psychoeducation may be required to help the family. It is important that the family have access to ongoing community support by the time they reach this stage.

The goal of the family intervention program in Calgary is to meet the needs of families based on this current research. Families are treated as collaborators in the treatment process. Each one is assigned a family worker who has special training in family work, and is solely dedicated to work with the family and integrate the family in the treatment plan. Individual family needs are assessed and interventions tailored (psychoeducation, communication and problem-solving training, and later on group work) to meet these needs. Family needs are re-assessed after six months, one year, two years, and at discharge (three years). These assessments will contribute to long-term analysis of the success of working with families from the time of onset of illness.

ALCOHOL/DRUGS AND RECOVERY

Recent research on the biological effects of substance use on a person with schizophrenia suggests that drugs or alcohol may have an effect on maintaining symptoms of psychosis, which in turn may have a neurotoxic effect on the brain. This could lead to irreversible change. This means that positive symptoms (see Chapter 3, Defining Positive and Negative Symptoms, p. 21) could actually increase or be exacerbated by use of drugs or alcohol, resulting in permanent damage to the brain. Studies have shown that up to sixty percent of people who suffer from schizophrenia either abuse or are dependent upon drugs and/or alcohol. Researchers are trying to understand the underlying reasons for this trend, and develop strategies to address it.

Common reasons given by people with schizophrenia for using alcohol and/or drugs include depression, anxiety, and negative side effects of antipsychotic medication. Ill individuals also report, however, that in reality the alcohol or drugs give them little relief from their symptoms. These findings suggest that treatment plans need to address complaints of depression, anxiety, and negative side effects of medication. Models for integrated treatment of people with schizophrenia who abuse substances have been developed and are being assessed for their effectiveness. One model in particular is sensitive to the different stages of schizophrenia. Its approach is persuasion, active treatment, and relapse prevention. Twelve-step programs, psychoeducation, social skills training, and support can be incorporated within these three treatment strategies. Participants learn about goal setting, reasons for relapses, high-risk situations, how to prevent relapses, how to manage finances, and the benefit of self-help activities. In a 1998 study of a group for individuals who participated in this integrated treatment strategy, it was found that after being involved in the group for one year (attending twice weekly sessions), forty-four percent of the participants no longer used alcohol or drugs. This evidence is very encouraging, and supports the use of integrated treatment programs.

Over the past few years, the Calgary EPP has been experimenting with an integrated approach to treatment for psychosis and substance abuse. Approximately thirty-seven percent of young people admitted to the program met the criteria for alcohol/drug abuse/dependence. The severity of the addiction is assessed at the initial assessment, again at the first year assessment, and re-assessed every three months for two years. Often times, ill individuals are not interested in EPP's specialty group (the Stopping Substances Group) when they are first admitted to the program. However, after one year in the program, EPP found there was a reduction in the number of ill people using alcohol or drugs, and a reduction in the level of use by those who continue to drink or use drugs. At the first year assessment, those individuals who still continue to abuse alcohol or drugs are presented with data that demonstrates their inability to stop drinking or using drugs. They are also presented with data that shows there has been no improvement in their symptoms, and told that a likely reason for this is alcohol or drugs. EPP has found that ill people who previously did not want to participate in the specialty group upon admission, are more willing to do so after being in the program for one year.

The goals of the Stopping Substances Group are as follows:

1)   To educate participants about current knowledge of the effects of drugs and alcohol, and the interaction of these substances with psychoses

2)   To develop commitment to reducing or abstaining from substance use

3)   To develop awareness of barriers to achieving these goals, and

4)   To learn and develop strategies to reduce or abstain from substance use

This special intervention group is comprehensive in context, using very detailed strategies to address the experiences of individuals with schizophrenia who also experience drug or alcohol problems.

THE CANADIAN BRAIN TISSUE BANK

As advances continue to be made in research laboratories throughout the

199

world, more and more people are beginning to appreciate the enormous potential of post-mortem human brain tissue research.

Although promising results are being reported and our understanding of severe neurologic and psychiatric disorders is improving, more significant progress is actually being delayed because of a scarcity of brain tissue donations.

The Canadian Brain Tissue Bank was established in 1981 in order to support medical research through the collection, storage, and distribution of brain tissue to interested scientific investigators. Such research is concerned with the causes, treatments and eventual cures for the many psychiatric and neurological disorders affecting so many people today. These include schizophrenia, Alzheimer's disease, dystonia, epilepsy, and many others. Research over the past decade has shown that the study of human brain tissue is essential to increasing our understanding of how the nervous system functions, and consequently in preventing and alleviating these illnesses. Most recently, post-mortem human brain research played a significant role in the development of a genetic test for Huntington's disease and a treatment for Parkinson's disease. Human brain tissue is also necessary because several serious neurologic and psychiatric conditions affect only humans and, therefore, animal models are not relevant. For comparative purposes, brain tissue is needed from healthy individuals, as well as from those who died with a neurologic or psychiatric illness.

There is also a critical need for relatives of people with genetically inherited disorders to donate their brains after death. Samples of DNA are kept from all tissue to help in future genetic testing.

APPENDIX A Glossary

Understanding The Language Of Mental Illness

If you have a relative, friend, or student with schizophrenia, you may find medical professionals and others using words you are not familiar with. This is a short glossary of some of the most commonly used terms.

Acute Dystonia

An extrapyramidal side effect, its symptoms include contraction of muscle groups, particularly the neck, eyes, and those muscles affecting posture. The individual may also experience discomfort, and an inability to think. Acute dystonia usually occurs within the first few hours of drug therapy.

Affective Disorders or Mood Disorders

Mental illness characterized by greatly exaggerated emotional reactions and mood swings from high elation to deep depression. Commonly used terms are manic-depression (or bipolar disorder) and depression
— although some people experience only mania and others only depression. These extreme mood changes are unrelated to changes in the person's environment.

Antipsychotics

Also referred to as neuroleptics or psychotropics, these are specific medications used in the treatment of mental illness, like schizophrenia. They are used to control psychotic symptoms such as delusions and hallucinations.

Delusion

A fixed belief that has no basis in reality. People suffering from delusions are often convinced they are famous people, are being persecuted, or are capable of extraordinary accomplishments.

Diagnosis

Classification of a disease by studying its signs and symptoms.

Schizophrenia is one of many possible diagnostic categories used in psychiatry.

Dyskinesia

This extrapyramidal side effect causes abnormal movements, such as: irregular blinking, grimacing, tongue movements and protrusion of the tongue, and worm-like movements of fingers and toes.

Electroconvulsive Therapy (ECT)

Used primarily for ill people experiencing extreme depression for long periods, who are suicidal, and who do not respond to medication or to changes in circumstances.

Extrapyramidal symptoms (EPS)

Side effects caused by antipsychotics. They include uncontrollable movements in the face, arms and legs. Parkinsonism, Acute dystonia, Dyskinesia, and Tardive dystonia are included in this group of symptoms. They can usually be managed by lowering the dose of the neuroleptic drug, adding or increasing the dose of an antiparkinsonian medication, or introducing other blocking drugs.

Hallucination

An abnormal experience in perception. Seeing, hearing, smelling, tasting or feeling things that are not there.

Involuntary Admission

The process of entering a hospital is called admission. Voluntary admission means ill persons request treatment, and are free to leave the hospital whenever they wish.

People who are very ill may be admitted to a mental health facility against their will, or involuntarily. There are two ways this can occur:

- Under medical admission certificates or renewal certificates

- Under special court orders when the person has been charged or convicted with a criminal offence. In this case, they may be held in a forensic facility

•	In some provinces, before someone can be admitted involuntarily under certificates, two physicians—one of whom is a psychiatrist —must certify that the person is: suffering from a mental disorder and requiring care, protection and medical treatment in hospital; unable to fully understand and make an informed decision regarding treatment, care and supervision; and/or likely to cause harm to self or others or to suffer substantial mental or physical deterioration if not hospitalized

Medications

In psychiatry, medication is usually prescribed in either pill or injectable form. Several different types of medications may be used, depending on the diagnosis. Ask your doctor or pharmacist to explain the names, dosages, and functions of all medications, and to separate generic names from brand names in order to reduce confusion.

1)	Antipsychotics: Brand Names—Modecate, Largactil, Stelazine, Haldol, Fluanxol, Piportil, Clozaril, Risperdal, Zyprexa. Generic Names— fluphenazine, chlorpromazine, trifluoperazine, haloperidol, flupenthixol, pipotiazine, clozapine, risperidone, olanzapine. These reduce agitation, diminish hallucinations and destructive behaviour, and may bring about some correction of other thought disorders. Side effects include changes in the central nervous system affecting speech and movement, and reactions affecting the blood, skin, liver and eyes. Periodic monitoring of blood and liver functions is advisable.

2)	Antidepressants: These are normally slow acting drugs — but if no improvement is experienced after three weeks, they may not be effective at all.

3)	Mood Normalizers: e.g., Lithium Carbonate, used in manic and manic-depressive states to help stabilize the wide mood swings that are part of the condition. Regular blood checks are necessary to ensure proper medication levels. There may be some side effects such as thirst and burning sensations.

4)	Tranquilizers: Valium, Librium, Ativan, Xanax, Rivotril. Generally referred to as Benzodiazepines. These medications can help calm agitation and anxiety.

5)	Side Effect Medications: Also called anticholinergics. Brand

Names— Cogentin, Kemadrin. Generic Names—benztropine, procyclidine.

Mental Illness/Mental Disorder

Physiological abnormality and/or biochemical irregularity in the brain causing substantial disorder of thought, mood, perception, orientation, or memory—grossly impairing judgement, behaviour, capacity to reason, or ability to meet the ordinary demands of life.

Mental Health

Describes an appropriate balance between the individual, their social group, and the larger environment. These three components combine to promote psychological and social harmony, a sense of well being, self-actualization, and environmental mastery.

Mental Health Act

Provincial legislation for the medical care and protection of people who are mentally ill. The Mental Health Act also ensures the rights of patients who are involuntarily admitted to hospital, and describes advocacy and review procedures.

Paranoia

A tendency toward unwarranted suspicions of people and situations. People with paranoia may think others are ridiculing them or plotting against them. Paranoia falls within the category of delusional thinking.

Parkinsonism

Another extrapyramidal side effect, Parkinsonism is divided into two categories: hypokinetic and hyperkinetic. Hypokinetic symptoms include decreased muscular movement, rigidity, awkward and stiff facial movements, and possibly depression and apathy. Hyperkinetic symptoms are agitation of lower extremities, agitation, tenseness, tremors, rapid rhythmic movements of the upper extremities. These symptoms commonly occur between a few days and a few weeks of treatment for an acute phase.

Psychiatrist

A physician that specializes in treating mental and emotional disorders.

Psychosis

Hallucinations, delusions, and loss of contact with reality.

Rehabilitation

Programs designed to help individuals return to normal functioning after a disabling disease, injury or addiction. They are designed to help people with mental illness live as independently as is possible.

Receptor

Special places on nerve cells that respond to specific chemical messages between cells.

Schizophrenia

Severe and often chronic brain disorder. Common symptoms—personality changes, withdrawal, severe thought and speech disturbances, hallucinations, delusions, and bizarre behaviour.

Side Effects

Side effects occur when there is drug reaction that goes beyond, or is unrelated to, the drug's therapeutic effect. Some side effects are tolerable, but some are so disturbing that the medication must be stopped. Less severe side effects include dry mouth, restlessness, stiffness, and constipation. More severe side effects include blurred vision, excess salivation, body tremors, nervousness, sleeplessness, tardive dyskinesia, and blood disorders.

Some drugs are available to control side effects. Learning to recognize side effects is important because they are sometimes confused with symptoms of the illness. A doctor, pharmacist, or mental health worker can explain the difference between symptoms of the illness and side effects due to medication.

Social Worker

A person specially trained to help individuals with social adjustment. A social worker would counsel persons with schizophrenia and their family on the social and emotional issues that arise from the disorder.

Tardive dystonia

One of the extrapyramidal side effects, recognized by unusual posture and dysarthria.

Treatment Plan

Refers to therapy or remedies designed to cure a disorder or relieve symptoms. In psychiatry, treatment is often a combination of medication, counselling (advice), and recommended activities. Together, these make up the ill individual's treatment plan.

Treatment Team (or Care Team)

Refers to the attending mental health professionals, case workers, etc. who work to provide services to the ill person in accordance with the treatment plan.

APPENDIX B   Further Resource Materials

Suggested Reading. The following books are highly recommended, and should be available through your local library or bookstore.

Adamec, Christine. How to Live with a Mentally Ill Person: A Handbook of Day-to-Day Strategies. John Wiley & Sons, 1996.

Appelbaum, Paul S. Almost a Revolution: Mental Health Law and the Limits of Change. Oxford University Press, 1994.

Amador, Xavier. I am not sick I don't need help. Vida Press Peconic, NY 2000.

Andreasen, Nancy C. The Broken Brain. Harper and Row, 1984.

Armat, Virginia C. & Isaac, Rael Jean. Madness in the Streets: How Psychiatry and the Law Abandoned the Mentally Ill. The Free Press, NY, 1990.

Backlar, Patricia. The Family Face of Schizophrenia. G.P. Putnam's Sons, New York, 1994.

Buckley, Peter F. & Waddington, J. Schizophrenia and Mood Disorders: The New Drug Therapies in Clinical Practice. Butterworth Heinemann, Boston, 2000.

Deveson, Anne. Tell Me I'm Here. Penguin Books, London, 1991. (Available in Libraries only.)

Gray, John E. & Shone, Margaret A. & Liddle, Peter F. Canadian Mental Health Law Policy. Butterworths Canada Ltd. Toronto, 2000.

Keefe, Richard & Harvey, D. Understanding Schizophrenia: A Guide to the New Research on Causes and Treatment. The Free Press, Macmillan, Toronto, 1994

Lafond, Virginia. Grieving Mental Illness: A Guide for Patients and Their Caregivers. University of Toronto Press, 1994.

Marsh, Diane T. & Dickens, Rex M. How to Cope with Mental Illness in Your Family: A Self-Care Guide for Siblings, Offspring, or Parents. Putnam, New York, 1997.

Mueser, Kim T. & Gingerich, Susan. <u>Coping With Schizophrenia: A Guide for Families</u>. New Harbinger, Oakland, CA, 1994.

Noble, K. & Lenz, S. <u>Children with Schizophrenia</u>. Glenrose Hospital Educational Services, Edmonton, Alta. 1995.

Secunda, Victoria. <u>When Madness Comes Home: Help & Hope for Children, Siblings, and Partners</u>. Disney Press, 1998.

**Torrey, E. Fuller. <u>Surviving Schizophrenia: A Manual for Consumers, Families, and Providers</u>. 3rd edition. Harper Collins, NY, 2001.

Woolis, Rebecca. <u>When Someone You Love Has a Mental Illness: A Handbook for Family, Friends, and Caregivers</u>. Putnam's Sons, New York, 1992.

EMERGENCY CONTACTS AND PHONE NUMBERS

Name:
_____

Number:

Name:
_____

Number:

Name:
_____

Number:

Name:
_____

Number:

Name:
_____

Number:

NOTES

NOTES

www.ingramcontent.com/pod-product-compliance
Lightning Source LLC
Chambersburg PA
CBHW021402210526
45463CB00001B/200